How Do We Know Who We Are?

How Do We Know Who We Are?

A Biography of the Self

~❧~

Arnold M. Ludwig

Oxford   New York
Oxford University Press
1997

Oxford University Press

Oxford   New York
Athens   Auckland   Bangkok   Bogotá   Bombay
Buenos Aires   Calcutta   Cape Town   Dar es Salaam
Delhi   Florence   Hong Kong   Istanbul   Karachi
Kuala Lumpur   Madras   Madrid   Melbourne
Mexico City   Nairobi   Paris   Singapore
Taipei   Tokyo   Toronto

and associated companies in
Berlin   Ibadan

Copyright © 1997 by Oxford University Press, Inc.

Published by Oxford University Press, Inc.,
198 Madison Avenue, New York, New York 10016

Oxford is a registered trademark of Oxford University Press

Library of Congress Cataloging-in-Publication Data
Ludwig, Arnold M.
How do we know who we are?: A biography of the self /
Arnold M. Ludwig.
p. cm.   Includes bibliographical references and index.
ISBN 0-19-509573-1
1. Man.   2. Self. (Philosophy)   I. Title.
BD450.L79   1997   126—dc20   96-23944

1 3 5 7 9 8 6 4 2

Printed in the United States of America
on acid-free paper

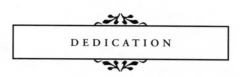

DEDICATION

For Ryan, Emily, Ellis, and Madeline
—With love, "Papaw"

CONTENTS

ACKNOWLEDGMENTS

T HIS BOOK HAS BEEN SHAPED by many influences. I owe a special
debt of thanks to all the distinguished biographers, historians, and writers
who generously agreed to be interviewed for this project and to share their time
and views with me. These individuals, in alphabetical order, are Christopher
Benfey, Victor Bockris, Alan Bullock, Humphrey Burton, James Collier, Louise
DeSalvo, Scott Donaldson, Leon Edel, Charles Bracelen Flood, Peter Gay, Brendan Gill, William Manchester, David McCullough, Diane Middlebrook, Joan
Peyser, Arnold Rampersad, Roxana Robinson, Donald Spoto, Wallace Stegner,
Gloria Steinem, and Linda Wagner-Martin. Sir Alan Bullock and Charles Bracelen Flood also were kind enough to review a chapter of the book in which they
had significant input.

Robert Straus, Guy Davenport, and John Ranseen critiqued and commented
on an earlier draft of the book. Gregory Guenthner, who has been my research
assistant over the years, contributed in so many ways to this project, including
editing my interviews with biographers, organizing files, reviewing chapters, and
a host of other activities. My wife, Aline, deserves particular thanks as both a critical sounding board for me and a constant source of inspiration during our frequent walks and talks. Last, my editor at Oxford, Joan Bossert, who was sup-
portive of this project ever since it was conceived, helped me to clarify my ideas,
made my writing more readable, and instructed me to be more tactful in my
remarks.

Trapped in an Epilogue

STANDING BEFORE A MIRROR, Friedrich Nietzsche apocryphally asked the deranged image staring back at him—"Who are you?"—and then repeated over and over again, "I am who I am." This may be the answer to the central question of human existence. Then, again, it may not.

Why write another book on the self? No matter what assumptions you make, you're likely to arrive at the same tautological conclusion as Nietzsche. You can't be other than what you are, unless of course, you believe that you can reinvent yourself or that your self is an illusion.

The reason I decided to write this book is that I had no choice. I had been composing it most of my life, only I didn't know it. In my clinical work, I found myself intrigued by my patients who were struggling to give voice to their "true" selves. As a scientist, I was drawn toward investigating the contortions of the self when people became psychotic or developed multiple personality or displayed overpowering cravings for drugs or were exposed to such powerful mind-altering techniques as hypnosis, sensory deprivation, or hallucinogens. And in my own personal life, I've always collected anecdotes about people from biographies, newspapers, magazines, films, and personal encounters, any tidbits that could shed light on who they were and what made them tick. All this, I tell myself, established my credentials as a *bona fide* expert on the self, perhaps not on the same plane as Plato, Aristotle, Kant, Descartes, and other famous philosophers who wrote brilliant treatises on this topic, but somewhere among the lesser lights who sometimes had trouble figuring out what these immortals had to say.

Why my lifelong interest in the self? I'm not sure, but I suspect it had some-thing to do with the manner of my conception. I never should have been born in the first place since I am the result of pseudocyesis, the medical term for a false pregnancy, which somehow always made me feel that my life was a disease or that my existence was unreal. According to my father, my parents were practic-ing a crude form of birth control when my mother miraculously became "preg-nant," complete with a swollen belly, enlargement of her breasts, and the absence of menses. After four months, when my father finally accepted the pregnancy as a *fait accompli*, he abandoned all forms of birth control, and it was then that I was conceived and born nine months later, after my mother's thirteen-month pregnancy.

The reason I'm writing this book now is that I can do so with a certain detachment. You see, by my calculations, after having lived a reasonably full life despite the manner of my conception, I should be dead now. At least, as a staunch believer in the genetic determinants of longevity, I lived a good part of my adult life expecting to die young. My father died of a heart attack at the age of fifty-two, and my mother died of cancer at the age of fifty-nine, so I had assumed that I never would live beyond the age of sixty. I lived my life accord-ingly, taking a final measure of myself during these past few years. Only here I am in my early sixties, healthy as far as I know, waiting for the telltale pang in my chest or the vague discomfort in my abdomen that I anticipated years ago. Though I continue to compose new chapters for my life story, they keep turning out as postscripts.

Perhaps if I could believe in an afterlife, I wouldn't be so preoccupied now with who I am and what life is all about. How comforting it would be to look forward to joining all my loved ones in heaven, as so many people look forward to joining theirs, except that I can't imagine what we'd talk about or do during our endless, incorporeal gatherings. The prospect of being with an omniscient God for eternity is no more attractive, since I always have been a bit of a loner and had trouble relating to people in authority. As for the pleasure I take in the extension of myself through my children and grandchildren, it's tempered by the knowledge that my genetic material will become progressively diluted, so that in five generations I'll only be one-thirty-second of myself, and in ten generations I may as well not have existed. Besides, I don't like the idea of sharing my progeny with so many strangers and having no say about who they are. So here I am, trapped in the epilogue between a completed life story that should not have happened and an afterlife I can't believe exists, and trying to make sense of both.

I have another confession to make. While this book is mine, it was a struggle to keep it so. Let me explain. Struck by how much we live our lives in biographical format, progressing from birth to childhood to adolescence to adulthood and to old age, I was inspired after my first couple of drafts to test out certain ideas on a skilled biographer or two and see if I could learn something more from them. After all, who should know better about the self than someone whose profession it is to reconstruct people from assorted information about them and, through the magic of the biographical process, give them the breath of life?

Who else to interview than the dean of modern biographers, Leon Edel, the author of the five-volume work on Henry James that required more than twenty years to complete and was the modern equivalent of James Boswell's biography of Samuel Johnson? But was he still alive? If so, he would be over ninety and probably suffering from the ravages of old age. After some detective work, I secured a phone number in Hawaii, called, and on the second ring, Edel himself answered, in a clear, firm voice that belied his age. My interview with him went so well that I decided to contact other biographers.

Leon Edel's name turned out to be a skeleton key for unlocking the door to many of the other biographers. One distinguished biographer after another agreed to be interviewed: William Manchester, Brendan Gill, David McCullough, Alan Bullock, Diane Middlebrook, Scott Donaldson, James Collier, Christopher Benfey, and Victor Bockris. The more I queried these individuals about their famous subjects and themselves, the more obsessed I became with my pursuit. The project took on a life of its own as I found myself tracking down other writers of well-known biographies: Gloria Steinem, Wallace Stegner, Peter Gay, Arnold Rampersad, Roxana Robinson, Joan Peyser, Linda Wagner-Martin, Humphrey Burton, Louise DeSalvo, Charles Bracelen Flood, and Donald Spoto. My collection of biographers soon swelled to twenty-one.[1] Only two writers turned me down, and one studiously ignored my written requests. My success rate was phenomenal, not because of my powers of persuasion but, I believe, because of the appeal of the topic itself. I began compiling a list of even more biographers to contact. But then I had a sobering insight—I had become hooked on this investigative process and had lost sight of its original purpose.

With this realization, I wrested myself away from the addictive pursuit, but I still wasn't able to break away entirely from the spell these biographers cast over me. When I undertook the next draft of my book, I found myself becoming an emcee for all the famous celebrities who were the subjects of their biographies—Marilyn Monroe, Winston Churchill, Laurence Olivier, Georgia O'Keeffe, Anne Sexton, Ernest Hemingway, Sigmund Freud, John F. Kennedy, Alfred Hitchcock, Leonard Bernstein, Adolf Hitler, Sylvia Plath, Langston Hughes, Arthur Ashe, John Cheever, Douglas MacArthur, Virginia Woolf, Theodore Roosevelt, Joseph Stalin, Harry S. Truman, Andy Warhol, and many others. I also served as a solicitous talk-show host for my collection of biographers, although I often disagreed with their views. This made interesting reading, but it wasn't the book I had planned to write.

It took two more drafts before I could reassert authorial control over my own manuscript. I decided to use excerpts from my interviews with these biographers to illustrate various points and, on occasion, as a basis for formulating and developing my own views. Although I believe I have succeeded reasonably well in matching these excerpts to the issues under discussion, I hope that I'll be forgiven when the fit is less than perfect. In these instances, I left the excerpts in because of their inherent interest.

Now a word about the contents of this book. The terrain of the self is vast, with parts known, parts impenetrable, and parts unexplored. As the first order of business, I examine what we know about the self and what we don't, and point out paradoxes about its properties—for instance, how a self can reflect upon itself, or deceive itself, or actualize itself, or be false. Adopting a narrative framework, which seems well-suited to a conceptualization of the self, I then discuss what it means to know ourselves or others, and whether it's possible for us to know anyone at all. Other issues I deal with are whether psychological truth is really true, whether sanity offers a better perspective of reality than madness, whether all personal identity is plagiarized, how people cope with the potential meaninglessness of their existence and the inevitability of their nonexistence, and whether personal authenticity is possible. I then address the crucial issue of whether we have the power to control our own lives, or whether all of our thoughts and actions are rooted in necessity.

Just as the task of a biographer is to fashion a man or woman out of his or her diaries, documents, dreams, memories, works, and assorted other materials, our task will be to form a coherent picture of the self from its many properties, paradoxes, and contradictions. Though interrelated, the chapters in the book can stand alone as essays, and don't necessarily have to be read in order. However, each of them fills in missing parts of a mosaic, and all are necessary to make the design clear. Viewed in its entirety, this mosaic reveals a new theory about the self, which has implications for who we are and what our existence is about.

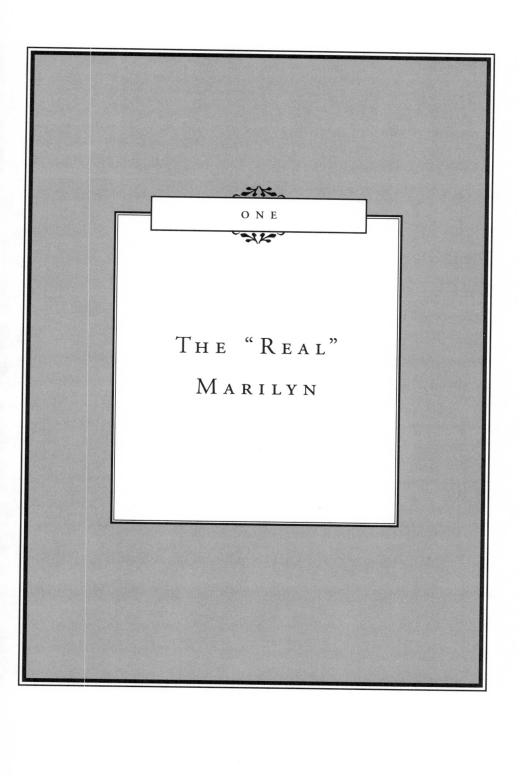

ONE

THE "REAL" MARILYN

ABOUT FIFTY BIOGRAPHIES or quasi-biographies have been written about Marilyn Monroe—more than about most famous statesmen, scientists, and creative artists of our time.[1] Why write so many biographies about one person? Five perhaps are understandable, maybe even ten. But fifty? Surely, there are other fascinating people to write about whose cultural achievements are far more important.

Part of the reason for this interest in Marilyn Monroe became clearer to me over the course of my reading twenty-five separate biographies about her, written mostly by people who should have known her well: former husbands, lovers, friends, fellow workers, admirers, and professional biographers or writers.[2] What emerged from my readings were different portraits of the actress, more varied than Andy Warhol depicted in his silkscreen photographs of her. Though these biographical portraits were intriguing, none, in my opinion, settled the mystery of who she was or why so many perceptive observers should see her so differently. But Marilyn Monroe apparently knew herself no better than those who tried to decipher her. "I seem to have a whole superstructure with no foundation, but I'm working on the foundation," she told reporters, and spent her life trying to do just that—to find herself.[3]

The first thing that caught my eye when I opened Gloria Steinem's book on Marilyn Monroe was her statement, "This is dedicated to the real Marilyn." And so I asked Steinem who that *real* person was.

"In her case, it was more clear and less subtle than it frequently is, because she clearly put on the persona of Marilyn," Steinem responded. "She would walk down the street unnoticed as herself and then say to her companion, 'I'll be Marilyn for a few minutes,' and then put on the mincing walk and the mannerisms and attract attention. People would recognize her as Marilyn. The distance between the little girl, Norma Jean, inside her, who had not been allowed to develop and who felt invisible, and the external Marilyn was very clear."

"Since you use the term 'real self' with Marilyn, how did you get to know what it was?" I persisted. "What categories of information did you use that other people didn't use?"

"I emphasized her childhood more than other writers did. Most of the writers have looked at her adult self and used it for sensationalism or felt sincerely that she must have desired these things or she wouldn't have done them. I tried to go back to her childhood and look at the ways it dictated the rest of her life."

"Would she have lost whatever personal magic she had if she had found this real self?"

"She might have lived, which of course is most important. The artificial self was the self that was doomed by age thirty or forty because it was a sex-goddess self. So there was no place for it to go. By all reports, she feared aging, almost more than death. So it seems to me that any persona that shortens your life is clearly artificial and going against your natural instincts toward health and survival. I think had she not been such a neglected child and felt invisible, she might have been less of a social stereotype, which might have made her less commercially successful. But it would have allowed her to play different kinds of roles. She hated being the dumb blonde."

"From what you know about her, did she buy into this public image of herself or did she have some personal sense of 'me'?"

"She clearly recognized that she could put on and take off her Marilyn persona. She clearly recognized that it was a separate persona. But she didn't seem to feel she was worthwhile without it, or she was too insecure to try to survive without it. . . . She believed she was invisible as a child. She only became visible [in the world] when she began to develop breasts and hips and be focused on by boys in a sexual way."

"Do you see her as a coherent self or many selves?"

"I see her as a coherent self who remained a child because the child never got what the child needed and because women in this culture are rewarded for being childlike. It was commercial. People looked at her and saw this vulnerability and malleability, since men are more trained to look for submission than cooperation in women. It was very sexual, though she herself said that she really didn't get sexual pleasure [and] turned to sex more for cuddling and security than for adult sexual pleasure."

"Many people put labels on themselves to define themselves. If you were defining her, what labels would you use?"

"Survivor, at least to a point. Obviously she didn't survive very long, but she struggled very hard. She had an enormous amount of strength, considering. . . . I guess, survivor and victim both."

"During a hypothetical conversation with her, you would have an opportunity to ask some unasked questions to help you fully understand her. What would you ask?"

"I don't know. My impulse is not so much to ask her as to offer help—to say, 'What you have gone through is an exaggerated version of what many women go through. I believe you about your sexual abuse. I believe you about everything you've ever said, and I support and honor your struggle, and you don't have to be Marilyn with me. You can say what you feel or be who you are.'"

"As a biographer, do you feel you know her better than she knew herself?"

"No, I probably didn't know her better than she knew herself. But I think that I liked her better than she liked herself."

Gloria Steinem's sympathetic portrayal of Marilyn Monroe seemed convincing to me at the time, but I also reacted similarly to the portrayals of many of her other biographers, each of whom interpreted her in entirely different ways. While I wasn't surprised that different biographers painted different portraits, I found it remarkable that some of these portraits seemed to be written about entirely different people, each with the same name. When I took all of these portraits into account, the composite picture that emerged was less one of a complex person than of a chimera, since it seemed improbable that someone should possess so many contradictory qualities.

The contrast between her Hollywood image as a sex symbol and her own perception of herself highlights some of these contradictions. No doubt this is a beautiful woman with an inviting mouth and glorious body, who revels in her sexuality, wantonly having affairs and parading about naked at parties, a femme fatale who breaks up marriages and whose clothed and unclothed poses serve as masturbatory fantasies for men throughout the world. Surely, much of what she did was deliberate, or so many people felt. But Marilyn Monroe had a different slant. "Admirers said it was my fault they wanted to kiss and hug me—it was the way I looked at them—I always felt they were talking about somebody else—I not only had no passion in me, I didn't know what it meant."[4] In one of her interviews, she said that for the longest time she would get as excited about sex as about a new stove polish. Despite her seeming sensuality, she seemed incapable of fully enjoying the act itself, rarely if ever having an orgasm. It may have been this lack of responsiveness on her part that prompted Tony Curtis, her co-star in the film *Some Like It Hot*, to tell reporters that kissing her was like kissing Hitler.

Obviously, Marilyn Monroe contributed to the confusion about her. With all her inconsistent responses to reporters over the years about her awful childhood, which could rival anything in a tale by Dickens, reality and fiction begin to merge. She says that when she was about eighteen months of age, she struggled to keep her deranged grandmother from smothering her with a pillow, but doesn't explain how an eighteen-month-old child could prevent it. She makes frequent mention of being an orphan, even though her mother was alive in a mental asylum, and she claims not to know who her father was, but by certain accounts she most likely did. She says she was sexually abused by a boarder at the age of eight, but the age and details change with the many retellings. She pleads to be taken seriously, but then informs us that she lived in her fantasies and that she exaggerated the orphan theme to Ben Hecht, who was writing a biography at the time, as a way to make her childhood more interesting to the public. Inconsistencies such as these likely prompted Norman Mailer, in his biography of Marilyn, to coin the term "factoids" to indicate facts that have no basis in reality, media creations that are not so much lies as attempts to manipulate the attitudes of the public.

To compound this confusion about her, the accounts of various biographers have transformed a seemingly obvious suicide in someone who made two prior attempts into a mysterious death. Now we find suggestions that she was murdered by the mob, the CIA, the FBI or people trying to protect the reputations of the President of the United States or his brother, Robert Kennedy, both of whom supposedly had affairs with her. Most recently, a distinguished biographer not only tried to dispel the commonly held belief that she was addicted to alcohol and pills but convincingly argued that the real culprit in her death may have been her psychiatrist, who told her housekeeper to administer a heavy dose of chloral hydrate through an enema, which then interacted adversely with the barbiturates already in her system.[5]

I asked Donald Spoto how he arrived at his distinctive image of Marilyn Monroe. "By a simple presentation of the truth," he responded, and continued: "That is to say, Marilyn Monroe was generally presented by people out for a quick buck. She has been presented as a woman of easy virtue, a drug addict, an alcoholic, self-destructive, suicidal, a weak and vulnerable person, utterly without discipline. None of this is true. She was not a drug addict. She was not an alcoholic. She was not a woman of easy virtue. She was not an unintelligent woman whose life was totally out of control. The facts simply will not support that very convenient myth which American people like very much to maintain, which goes like this: A beautiful, sexy, blonde woman must be a tramp. And if she wasn't, we'll force people to believe that she was, simply make up some stories to believe that she was. So we issue her Kennedy as her lover. We issue her wild numbers of people with whom she had sexual relationships. There's no connection to the truth. The biographer simply tells the truth. That's how my book differs from those that have preceded. It simply tells the truth about her life."

"Do you feel that she had problems with her identity? Was she struggling to find out who she was? I'm asking, too, whether you believe there is such a thing as an authentic self?"

"I don't see self and identity as static givens which exist like platonic forms, which a person may discover and impose on himself. I see identity and self as realities in process. To be one's self . . . simply means to close the gap between who one claims to be in a celebrity famished society and who one was in the process of becoming. . . . It's extremely difficult for anyone so much in the public eye to have the time and space and quiet to find out precisely what is going on in the deepest recesses of the soul. . . . (Marilyn Monroe) engaged upon this with extraordinary success. She did remarkably well given the roles she had in the fifties. I don't mean the movie roles, but the role that was imposed on her as a sex goddess."

Who is this mysterious person who defies characterization and can generate so much conjecture and disagreement not only among people who knew her well but also among trained, scholarly biographers? Which of these many portraits, if any, captures the real Marilyn Monroe? Marilyn Monroe herself gives us an important clue about the reason for her many portrayals. "The truth is I never fooled anyone," she said. "I've let men sometimes fool themselves. . . . They would invent a character for me. . . . They were loving someone I wasn't. When they found out, they would blame me for disillusioning them and fooling them."[6]

What she is saying, then, is that she often doesn't set out to create the impression others have of her, but that others, because of their own needs, project certain qualities on her. She seems justified in her observation, but perhaps not completely so. Though her image tends to mirror others' expectations of her, much like Woody Allen's *Zelig*, it's sometimes hard to tell how much she herself unwittingly encourages their expectations.

"There have been many biographies done of Marilyn Monroe," I remarked to Wallace Stegner. "As a biographer, novelist, and writer, how would you go about judging who Marilyn Monroe was when you have all these different versions? What criteria would you use?"

"I guess I look for as many signs as I can find of objectivity or a willingness to see the whole picture, for as few signs as I can find of delusion or illusion. Marilyn Monroe, after all, is a character that is hard to look at . . . for many males, particularly, maybe females, too . . . without illusion. Anybody who writes a biography of somebody like that is going to find the things in her that he's unconsciously looking for.

"Once when I was fooling around in New York doing something or other," he continued, "I went into the Art Students League. I was looking for somebody, and I wandered into a life class and found myself embarrassingly standing around talking to some people by this naked woman who was posing. She was a very striking black girl, a real Amazon, a beautiful woman. I looked at some of the pictures that six or eight art students were making. One of these people was a Japanese, one was black, two or three were white males, one was a white woman. From the pictures that I saw of that statuesque, black girl on their easels, I could have identified the painter without knowing who painted it. The Japanese one made her look somehow Japanese. The black girl accentuated her blackness. The white males accentuated her voluptuousness. And it would have made a nice object lesson. I think that happens in writing as well."

How, then, do we go about establishing which version of Marilyn Monroe among the many available is most authentic? What criteria should we use to get beyond her public facade? Perhaps the biographers themselves, experts on the construction of character, can provide insights on this matter. I took a sampling of twelve of the twenty-one biographers I interviewed and got twelve different answers. There were, though, some overlapping emphases.

Certain biographers placed great importance on the credentials of those creating the portraits and whether they had a sufficient range of experience to draw from to have empathy for their subject. Others pointed to the reliability of the available information and the existence of credible, eyewitness accounts. A couple stressed the need for information about the kind of nurturing the subject was exposed to during childhood. One said that any valid portrayal had to explain why Marilyn acted as she did. Several biographers said that the most convincing portrait was one that best captured her quiddities and most telling gestures. A couple argued that no biography could be authentic because they all were based on partial truths. And one biographer insisted that each of her many biographies represented some aspect of the real Marilyn, since she was a kaleidoscopic combination of different persons: professional, domestic, and maternal.

Add to these different perspectives the abbreviated comments offered by the two biographers of Marilyn Monroe in my sample. Gloria Steinem said that unlike the approach of Norman Mailer, who assumed Monroe was lying about much of what she said, even her childhood sexual abuse, a realistic portrayal must start with Monroe's own words. The biographer needs to give credence to what she says, but naturally, in the context of her actions. Donald Spoto's emphasis was more scholarly. He mentioned the importance of looking at the end of the biography to see if there is "a critical apparatus," which includes source notes, acknowledgments, a listing of the people interviewed, and the archives used, because information of this sort tells us whether the biographer did his homework or instead was advancing his own agenda.

DECODING PEOPLE

Where do all these expert opinions leave us? Hoping to find some nuggets of biographical truth in my brief survey, I was at first discouraged by these seemingly contradictory perspectives. Although there was some overlap among these opinions, they were as diverse as the many portraits of Monroe. Any biographer's portrayal of her could be as realistic as that biographer believed it to be and as unconvincing as any other biographer, using different standards, saw it. Did this mean there could be no accurate or definitive portrait of a person?

Despite these seemingly different responses, there was at least one point about which almost all the biographers in my limited survey agreed. Regardless of their personal perspectives, they emphasized the need for reliable information and, as much as possible, an objective interpretation of it—although each biographer assigned different weights to different categories of information and tended to interpret this information differently. Still, this was an important starting point. What we need to explore now is what type of information about a person is most important, how to ensure its reliability, and whether it's possible to examine it through unbiased lenses.

Using my extensive interviews with biographers as a springboard, I identified four main sources of information that contribute to our opinions about others.[7] One source is obviously what people say. Another involves the experiences they share with others. Another is their behavior. Yet another source has to do with what they produce or create. Would a composite of all these sources of information give a complete and objective picture of a person? Not necessarily so if this information is incomplete, flawed, or distorted.

THE SPOKEN WORD

The first question we need to ask is, what stock should be placed on what people reveal about themselves in conversations, interviews, correspondences, or memoirs? Much of what we know about Marilyn Monroe comes from information of this sort: her personal autobiography, countless interviews with the press, and personal observations she made to others. Yet the reliability of many of these revelations may be difficult to establish.[8]

The autobiography, *Marilyn Monroe: My Story*, offers us a problem even before we open it, since it supposedly represents the true confessions of a make-believe person, a Hollywood creation.[9] She was born Norma Jean Mortensen. She isn't "Marilyn Monroe", her stage name, or is she? In her book she treats Norma Jean Mortensen mostly metaphorically, but sometimes as almost a separate entity within her. For instance, before getting ready to go out, she describes giving Norma Jean a treat in the bath; then, after getting out of the tub, spending a long time rubbing creams into her skin; and finally putting on her clothes as slowly as she can, because "the later I am the happier Norma Jean grows."[10] She reveals this about herself, but it's hard to know what she is revealing.

Then there is the vague and varying account of a boarder who made her undress when she was eight or nine and touched her in an unspecified way. Though the substance of her allegation is likely to be true, she may be embroidering it for dramatic effect. She openly admits that becoming a great performer is the mission of her life. "At thirteen," she writes, "when I put on my bathing suit for the first time, I knew I belonged to the public and the world—Public was the only family, Prince Charming and the only home I dreamed of."[11] If there is any truth in Norman Mailer's claim that she lived in a continuing condition of a half-lie, which she imposed on everyone as an absolute truth, then we're faced with the well-known philosophical conundrum of whether an inveterate liar is telling the truth when he says he is lying.[12]

Yet in all fairness, autobiographical materials do offer important information about persons. When Marilyn reveals that "The men I find I'm most attracted to are those least capable of making me happy," [13] or that she used to playact all the time because, "It meant I could live in a more interesting world than the one around me,"[14] her confessions have the ring of truth—they're consistent with other information we know about her.

The difficulty with autobiographical accounts, memoirs, personal communications, or self-reports of all kinds is that they are by their very nature subjective. People see the world through their own eyes and have a vested interest in their perceptions. Any personal accounts of their lives or attempts to explain what they think, feel, and do involve interpretations on their part, which usually tend to be self-serving. In the case of celebrities who hope to create a certain public image, facts and fiction often become indistinguishable. James Collier, who has interviewed many musical greats as part of his biographical research, informs me that most celebrities develop canned interview responses, which, after many repetitions, they come to believe. "In show business," he says, "you have the problem of always dealing with the act, dealing with the star, as opposed to the person. One of the big problems is trying to scrape that away, but usually they're too smart for you. . . . Great chunks of these canned biographies get to be believed by these people. They're much nicer things to believe than what really happened."

Aside from their biased perspective, autobiographical accounts also tend to suffer from selective and faulty recollections. Despite the common notion that our mind functions like a video camera, faithfully recording all our experiences, (which, if forgotten, may become accessible through psychotherapy, dreams, or hypnosis), recent research suggests otherwise. It appears that our actual memories change over time, and that we tend to "reconstruct" rather than "recover" them as details fade or become lost. In short, we automatically seem to be remolding our past to fit our present circumstances or emotional needs and to maintain a consistent personal narrative. Because these altered or fabricated recollections convey the same sense of emotional conviction and realness as accurate memories, we never may be able to establish their validity, no matter how vivid they seem.

Inspired by his famous novel *Angle of Repose*,[15] in which the protagonist recounts his life almost in autobiographical fashion, I asked Wallace Stegner his views about the nature of autobiography. "I have a kind of strange feeling about autobiography," he replied. "Once, half a dozen years ago, somebody asked me to write a short, ten thousand word autobiography for some reference book, which I did, and I discovered two or three things while writing it. One was that I wasn't to be trusted with autobiography because I kept wanting to correct things as I went along and make it turn out more on my side, make myself look better. For another thing, I had a feeling that I had written it all before, because so many of the things in my autobiography, in some way or other, had been used in my fiction. I think a lot of novelists have a tendency to write their autobiographies obliquely in fiction. I don't know of that many great autobiographies by fiction writers. Statesmen seem to go in for that more than we do. But I'm sure that we are slyly revealing ourselves in a way we want to be revealed when we write an autobiography and we probably are protecting ourselves in places where we feel we need protection. I wouldn't doubt that for a minute."

Pursuing this observation, I asked, "Do you believe that it's possible for a person to invent himself or herself through autobiographical accounts, or is the basic person going to show through in some way?"

"Well, people have invented themselves, public characters for themselves, invented whole careers, biographies, actions, names even, relatives. Katherine Anne Porter was a famous case in point. She invented a whole childhood for herself. The whole career of her youthful escapades, marriages, and so on, most of it was invented. And she wrote stories that were apparently transparent reflections of her own autobiographical experience, which when you examine them in terms of the facts of her life, as far as they're detectable, turn out to have been sly fictions. So she could be said to have invented her character, her past, her relationships, the whole business. Her whole life in effect was a fiction. Some people would say a lie, but I think it was fairer to say a fiction."

What Stegner intimated but didn't say was that the extent of Porter's fabrications far exceeded anything she allowed the characters in her fiction to do. According to her biographer, Porter edited the story of her life as she might have rewritten one of her short stories, selecting or inventing events that best suited her plot. As she reshaped her past, the more acceptable version became her new truth. She herself was to confess, "My own habit of writing fiction has provided a wholesome exercise to my natural, incurable tendency to try to wrangle the sprawling mess of our existence in this bloody world into some kind of shape." [16]

SEEING THROUGH OTHERS' EYES

Whatever reservations we have about the reliability of public disclosures presumably should be put to rest with the personal information we acquire during intimate encounters, personal confessions, or shared experiences, the kinds of encounters that potentially take place between lovers, a caring parent and a trusting child, a penitent and a priest, close friends, or a patient and therapist—the kinds of encounters that take place when people's guards are down and they reveal their innermost thoughts, feelings, and dreams. This kind of information involves not only verbal communications but nonverbal experiences as well, such as sexual encounters, watching a sunrise together, sharing an ordeal, or even taking a shower together. We gather this information about others largely through "empathic identification"—the ability to wear others' skin, walk in their shoes, or see through their eyes; or through "vicarious introspection"—the ability to imagine how they actually think and feel. [17]

What are a few of the insights about Marilyn Monroe that people who knew her intimately reveal in their biographical accounts? Since she represents a sex symbol, let's hear about her own sexual proclivities. A photographer, who supposedly discovered her and refers to their relationship as little more than friends and little less than lovers, reveals that her sexual appetites exceeded his ability to give her pleasure. Supposedly, she also was never more relaxed than when preening and admiring herself while naked in a sort of dreamy trance before a full-length mirror. [18] A self-described lover and friend for over twenty years says that Marilyn would go out and pick up guys in a bar and then, after sex, tell them they "fucked" Marilyn Monroe, and take pleasure from the expression on their faces. Another biographer says that when she had a man in bed, she didn't need sleeping pills. Her first husband described her as an uncomplicated, happy, domestic housewife. Arthur Miller, her last husband, claimed that she was "sometimes on her knees before her own body and sometimes despairing because of it." [19]

These selective perceptions by some of those intimate with her offer a confusing picture about her sexuality. Descriptions range from that of a domestic housewife to a lover with insatiable sexual needs to a wanton woman who randomly picked up men at bars. How do we reconcile these observations by intimates with seemingly conflicting evidence? By her own admission, she was "as unresponsive as a fossil" to sexual advances and hardly ever had an orgasm. And at least one distinguished biographer denied that she was promiscuous. Of course, we could dismiss some of these reports as "trash," as I have heard certain of my interviewees do, but this still wouldn't eliminate all the inconsistent observations among other people who knew her well.

The limitation of information gained from close encounters or empathic understanding, convincing as it may be, is that it's based entirely on how we interpret what others reveal and what they do, or how we imagine they must feel. We make assumptions without proof. Even when we supposedly share the same experience with others, we never can be sure that their experiences are the same as ours. Though it makes intuitive sense to assume a universality of human experience, that what we and others feel in a given circumstance must be the same, intuitive sense isn't necessarily true. One difference in a shared experience, for instance, is that others (and whatever personal meaning they have for us) are part of our experience, while we (and whatever personal meaning we have for them) are part of theirs. Therefore, while the assumption of a shared, identical experience is reasonable, it can't be logically true.

Another problem with empathic understanding is its evanescent nature. With this type of knowing, what we know about others can change drastically, depending on time and place and circumstance. Lovers who once knew each other so well and had such wonderful rapport can become strangers and even adversaries when love is gone. Once close friends and confidantes have a misunderstanding and then drift apart. The wonderful camaraderie established between drinking buddies or pot smokers often disappears when the intoxication wears off. Or therapists who believe they know their patients so well may often be unaware of their deceptions.

DO ACTIONS SPEAK LOUDER THAN WORDS?

People not only impart information about themselves through personal accounts, but also through their behavior. Actions are supposed to speak louder than words. The viewpoint of the strict behaviorist is that anything meaningful about people rests in their behavior, which is both objective and measurable, and not in their experience, which is subjective and unprovable. While this argument has its merits, it also has its drawbacks, especially so when applied to Marilyn Monroe.

Take, for example, the many conflicting observations of her behavior by people who supposedly knew her well. One source portrays her to be as naive and forthright as an ingenue; another as careless with the truth. One source describes her as a victim of men and the system; another as an exploiter of both. One source describes her as lacking in common sense and mindlessly stupid; another as smart, manipulating, even calculating. One source describes her as fragile, insecure, and needy; another as strong and determined. One source describes her as a giving, caring person who wore her heart on her sleeve; another as petty, bitchy, vindictive, and cruel. One source describes her as spontaneous and alive; another as always having the aura of death about her. One source describes her as a pitiful, beaten creature with no self-esteem; another as a supreme narcissist who almost makes love to herself in the mirror. One source claims that she is interested in self-discovery; another that she never told her various psychiatrists the full truth. These contradictions go on and on.

Despite the different ways of interpreting the same behavior, behavior represents an important source of information about people. By definition, it is how they behave. But the ways people behave don't necessarily reflect what they think or feel and what may be special about them. Their public behavior can be just as misleading as the attitudes or opinions they express, and sometimes more so. Society's constraints on what is proper, decent, desirable, and safe are far greater on public acts than private thoughts. Actions can be observed and censured; thoughts cannot. For that reason, what others do at times may be less a direct reflection of their underlying motivation than an expedient disguise for their private fantasies and thoughts.

IS THE POEM THE POET?

If social behavior can be misleading, perhaps for a creative artist such as Marilyn Monroe we should rely less on her statements or public persona and more on her artistic productions. Many believe this is the most meaningful information about people since it reveals the highest expression of their selves. Supposedly, through creative activity—whether art, music, dance, architecture, acting, improvisation, decorative arrangements, woodwork, writing—they display their unique sensibilities and perceptions and any unresolved conflicts as well.

Among my biographer informants, many relied on the fiction, movies, art, or music produced by their subjects as one of the main ways of gaining insights about them and interpreting who they were. Leon Edel, for instance, informed me that if his subject is a literary person, a writer, he reads his or her words "because that tells me almost everything I want to know." For Marilyn Monroe, we would have to search for her distinctive qualities in movies such as *Gentlemen Prefer Blonds, How to Marry a Millionaire,* or *Some Like It Hot,* or later, in *The Misfits,* a movie written by her husband at a time when their marriage was breaking up. What of significance could we learn about her by examining these films? Aside from her comedic gifts, we would note the image she conveys of a beckoning vulnerability and innocent sexuality, along with her rare combination of girlish naiveté and female shrewdness. This may help us explain her behavior off screen and the response of others to her, too. Her appearance and manner could explain why almost all the men who were attracted to her, aside from their more lascivious motives, felt bound to help her "grow up"—wanting her to be more domestic, to improve her mind, or to become a more serious actress—and could also explain her initial need to please them, and then her later resentment about doing so.

No doubt, the creative works of people tell us much about their talent and genius and often the themes that attract them, but in Marilyn's case, biographers might have to stretch their imaginations to tell much about her from her films, other than her ability to exercise her personal magic and act her usual roles off screen as well as on. We know that she can play the dumb, sexy blonde to perfection, but because she was mostly typecast for this role, we don't know the full range of other roles that might suit her.

Unfortunately, there are certain conceptual problems in relying on creative works to tell us about creative people. One problem has to do with the assumption that creative expression necessarily reveals something fundamental about a subject's character. No doubt, in many instances, people strive to communicate their personal visions in their works. But in other instances, they may choose to mislead the public or hide behind their art. This often is so in actors or musical

performers, many of whom only seem to find an identity on stage or while enact-
ing certain roles.

Another problem has to do with the distinctive properties of the different
media of expression. Usually, what we can learn about writers from their works
is different from what we can learn about artists, architects, musicians, or actors
from theirs. Nonverbal forms of expression may not be readily translatable into
verbal forms. Creative artists themselves may not be able to explain the basis of
their inspiration, or may interpret their own works differently from most
informed critics. They also may give voice to what they imagine other people
experience or feel.

Perhaps the most basic problem in judging people from their works is of a
logical nature. Though people may try to express themselves through their writing, music, acting, or art, their works must stand largely on their own. Their personal attributes may have nothing to do with their works. An insensitive, immature person may compose a magnificent symphony. An otherwise sensitive,
mature person can create a trite, flawed painting. A philosopher or poet may celebrate humanity and Nature in his writings yet appear to all the world as a mis-
anthrope. It's fallacious to equate people with their works because we use entirely
different criteria to evaluate life and art. Still, that doesn't keep most biographers
from doing so. The problem is that they often have little other intimate information about their subjects to rely on.

I asked Wallace Stegner, "To what extent do you think it's legitimate to
look at the works of somebody, the writings, the fiction, and to extrapo-
late from them to the person? If someone was writing a biography of
you, could he tell from your writings about you or would your writings
be like a Rorschach for him?"

He answered: "With one kind of novelist, say a Hemingway, you
can tell quite a lot about him simply by the characters he draws, most of
which are clones of himself. That kind of writer, the kind we call subjective, writes hardly veiled autobiography. I do some of that myself.
Sure there are all kinds of clues to character in there, but it's protective,
too. It's done with the kind of cunning that novelists acquire. They're all
ventriloquists and shape-shifters and they have protective coloration, so
that it's not by any means the most accurate way of getting at the char-

acter of the biographer or the novelist. I think something unprotected like letters is a much safer source."

COMPOSING A COMPOSITE

As an exercise, let's recap some of what we know about Marilyn Monroe. A thumbnail sketch, organized under different headings, is all that's necessary to make a point.

Fear of Abandonment. Marilyn Monroe began her life emotionally disadvantaged. Her maternal grandparents had been in mental institutions, her uncle committed suicide, and her mother was in and out of mental hospitals for a good part of her life. Add to this family legacy of insanity that she spent time in about ten foster homes, two years in the Los Angeles Orphan Home, then four years with an appointed guardian, and never had a relationship with her father, and it seems she had more than sufficient grounds to fear abandonment by those who mattered most to her.

Identity Disturbances. Much of Marilyn Monroe's sense of identity seemed grounded in her body. This focus undoubtedly became sharpened sometime in her early teens when she discovered she was physically attractive to men. As with almost anyone growing up who discovers she has a special gift that elicits attention and approval, she developed and exploited it, and sought out settings in which it could be best expressed, such as on-screen or in the bedroom. The rich, the mighty, and the famous worshipped at the altar of her body, and she did, too. But she had her doubts. Beauty has an evanescent quality, and in time begins to fade. So she spent increasing amounts of time keeping up her appearance, trying to reassure herself before the ever-present mirror that she was still the fairest maiden of them all. Not surprisingly, this didn't satisfy her. Did she see the most beautiful woman in the world or the insecure Norma Jean staring back at her? She sought to solidify her shaky sense of self through psychotherapy and by throwing herself into different roles: housewife, intellectual, or Jewish convert. Even in her search for authenticity, she still seemed to be playing a role. She was Marilyn Monroe, a make-believe Hollywood creation, paradoxically trying to find her real self by playing the part that self-seekers were supposed to act: reading deep books, getting psychoanalyzed, and speculating a lot about who she really was.

Pattern of Unstable and Intense Relationships. Part of the Monroe mystique involves the legion of famous and not-so-famous men with whom she had sexual relationships. Her life was marked by the glow of love affairs that sometimes led to tumultuous marriages and the bitterness and despair that came when they finally collapsed. Many of those she initially admired she later grew to hate.

Emotional Instability. All during her adult life, Marilyn Monroe showed mood swings, shifting from moments of joy and happiness to the depths of desperation and gloom. Almost everyone who knew her was aware of her quicksilver moods. At times she could be businesslike and professional, and then suddenly become immature, demanding, and impetuous.

Inappropriate and Difficult-to-Control Anger. Her sudden rages, fury, and hysterics on and off the movie set became legendary. But then, just as rapidly, she could become pleading or irresistibly sweet. Sometimes, her transformations from being reasonably calm and poised to being foul-mouthed, angry, and irrational shocked her friends and colleagues. Laurence Olivier, who once worked with her on a movie, attributed these changes to her being "schizoid." Having once been doused with a glass of champagne by Monroe, Tony Curtis, her co-star in *Some Like It Hot,* spoke later of her being viciously arrogant and vindictively selfish.

Self-Damaging Impulsiveness. Along with her rapid mood changes and at times flashflood anger, Marilyn Monroe also showed signs of being impetuous and impulsive. Aside from her numerous sexual encounters and sometimes provocative displays of nakedness, she indulged in substance abuse. Plagued by chronic insomnia, she often would become desperate for sleeping pills and periodically take enormous quantities of them. At times she tried to inveigle sleeping pills from friends and pleaded with her doctors and psychiatrists for drugs to calm her nerves and help her sleep. Her many "collapses" on the movie set and subsequent hospitalizations, which usually brought production to a halt, were attributed to her excessive alcohol and drug use.

Transient Alterations in Awareness. Aside from her frequent intoxications, Marilyn Monroe also was prone to other forms of altered awareness. When she sometimes treated Norma Jean almost as another person, she seemed to be dissociating and showing a splitting of her self. She also displayed self-induced trance states. Before each take on the movie set for *Some Like It Hot,* for instance, she would close her eyes and enter a deep trance, "then suddenly start to flail her hands violently, up and down, up and down, as if she were desperately intent upon separating her hands from her wrists."[20]

Chronic Feelings of Emptiness. Despite her many talents and successes, Marilyn Monroe remained unhappy and discontented. She herself commented on her lack of any personal foundation and her defective sense of self. One of her secretaries observed that she was "the emptiest human being I ever encountered." She seemed to have a bottomless need for love, which often elicited a caring response from the men in her life. Her terrible loneliness and neediness seemed to be almost too much for her psychiatrists. Responding to her insatiable need for attention, her last psychiatrist inappropriately invited her to live with him and his family and for a period of time saw her for four or five hour sessions almost every day.

Recurrent Suicidal Behavior. With her chronic unhappiness and her unquenchable emotional needs, Marilyn Monroe often flirted with suicide. Before the age of nineteen, she already had made two suicide attempts, one with gas and the other with sleeping pills. This preoccupation with suicide surfaced many times over the years. Because of their concern for her, several people close to her got her to agree to suicide pacts, whereby if she ever seriously thought of killing herself, she would call them first, and vice versa. Among the many biographies written about her are references to periodic drug overdoses, which likely represented suicide gestures or attempts. Then, in her final act, at the premature age of 36, she took (or was administered) an overdose of chloral hydrate and ended her remarkable and tragic life.

Now let's pause a moment and review what we've done. Based on our selection and interpretation of the various sources of information about Marilyn Monroe, we've created an ersatz biography of her. But this isn't an unusual exercise. Even though we don't do so formally, we can't help constructing mental biographies, sometimes lengthy but mostly abbreviated ones, about the people we know or wish to know. It's part of the process of knowing them. Though lacking many details, we need to fit whatever information we have about them into a comprehensible and convincing life story that conforms to the biographical format.

Is our extrapolated biographical portrait of Marilyn Monroe any more or less accurate than those of people who actually met her, worked with her, lived with her, or interviewed those who did? It's hard to say. It certainly isn't as scholarly, as comprehensive, or as thoughtful as most, but that may not make any difference. That's because there is no way to prove one biographical interpretation of her to be truer than another. Our makeshift, admittedly skimpy biography, which rearranges the observations of others and gives certain of these observations different emphases, is simply another version. If fifty versions of her existed before, now there are fifty-one, this one shaped by the information about her I chose to include and the particular ways I interpreted it. This raises the question whether a person's self can exist independently of others' perceptions, or whether it needs others' perceptions to give it dimension and form.

In the case of Marilyn Monroe, we have a kaleidoscope of different perceptions about her, many of which seem to reflect the value judgments or personal attitudes of the perceivers. Words like bitchy, controlling, confused, generous, conceited, lost, fragile, critical, sweet, calculating, wanton, innocent, trusting, vindictive, vulnerable, tough, unpredictable, and helpless, which provide the coloring and brush strokes for Monroe's various portraits, aren't objective qualities, such as height, weight, or eye color, but are personal interpretations about her by people who either like her, are sympathetic toward her, resent what she symbolizes, or have personal axes to grind. Certain of these interpretations are more skillful, artful, imaginative, and insightful portrayals of her than others, but each brings its own distinctive perspective into play.

Can we ever know someone photo-realistically and objectively? Biographers themselves disagree on the extent to which this can be done. At one end of the continuum of opinions, some believe that personal biases can be reduced through careful scholarship, archival documentation, and corroboration of facts, or even, as Scott Donaldson, borrowing a phrase from Hemingway, put it, by having a good "shit detector." At the other end of the continuum, other biographers frankly admit that they never can escape their biases. Louise DeSalvo, the biographer of Virginia Woolf, for instance, claims that objectivity isn't possible in biography, and even if it was, empathy for the subject is more important, as long as the biographer openly states her biases. In an article, Sharon O'Brien, the biographer of Willa Cather, puts the matter most bluntly. "The biographer's objectivity is a myth," she writes. "Emotional and psychological currents that we do not fully understand draw us to our subjects; if we are lucky, we do not lose either ourselves or our subjects in the resulting whirlpool."[21]

Another issue needs comment. Perhaps there are some readers who have divined my surreptitious intention in organizing my impromptu biographical portrayal of Marilyn Monroe as I did. If so, they will have detected that the headings for each of the paragraphs within this makeshift account (i.e., "fear of abandonment," "emotional instability," "identity disturbances," and so on) represent the actual diagnostic criteria for a borderline personality disorder, as represented in the official *Diagnostic and Statistical Manual of Mental Disorders, Fourth Edition*, published by the American Psychiatric Association.[22] To qualify for this diagnosis, the person must meet at least five of the total of nine criteria listed. As we've seen, Monroe clearly meets all nine.

So now, instead of a puzzling, mysterious person with contradictory qualities, about whom people seem to disagree, we have someone familiar to most mental health workers. Her very unpredictability, mood swings, neediness, shifts from idealizing people to devaluing them, and self-destructiveness can even become highly predictable. These behaviors make her and the many others like her extremely difficult, frustrating patients for therapists. Her last psychiatrist, for instance, who clearly became overinvolved in her care, later wrote, "I had become a prisoner of a form of treatment that I thought was correct for her, but almost impossible for me. At times I felt I couldn't go on with this."[23]

But now look what we've done. By focusing on the interpretive labels instead of the simple descriptions of her behavior, we've transformed our ersatz biography of her into a case study. As with the well-known illusion, in which the face of an attractive, young woman becomes transformed into an old hag's, by a blink of our eyes we've likewise changed Marilyn Monroe from a beautiful, talented, but temperamental young woman into a very disturbed mental patient. Her personal magic disappears, and presto, she becomes her disease.

Now how exactly did this transformation come about? It came about in almost the same way that the different biographies or portrayals of her came about, or for that matter, the same way that different people manage to see any particular person differently. Because of my training and background—my inclinations, if you will—I chose to see whether a comprehensive psychiatric diagnosis could parsimoniously account for Monroe's seemingly contradictory behaviors. And of course, it did, amazingly so at first glance . . . but not surprisingly so for me. The reason I wasn't surprised that she fit this diagnosis so well was that I knew she would; this is because I arbitrarily selected it beforehand from the array of psychiatric diagnoses others had given her. Then, to dramatically make a point about how our prior biases can shape and distort our perceptions of others, I deliberately presented only information about her that supported this diagnosis and excluded other information that contradicted it.

Whether this diagnosis actually is correct, I have no way of knowing since I didn't examine her personally and didn't have access to all the facts.[24] Yet even if it is true, something bothers me about seeing her in this pathological way. The diagnosis captures Marilyn Monroe, but her essence disappears. Like a butterfly impaled on a display board, she becomes a lifeless form. By resorting to a taxonomy and putting clinical labels on her behavior, we've taken away her uniqueness. She actually may meet the criteria for a borderline personality disorder, but she is much more than any clinical diagnosis.

The mystery remains about who the real Marilyn is. Parts of her may be scattered among the fifty-odd biographies about her, but as we've seen, we can't tell which are most vital and whether they add up to a whole. None of the biographies is definitive, and now we must admit that even a possible clinical diagnosis that accounts for much of her behavior doesn't adequately depict her. Should we then despair of ever knowing her or, for that matter, any other human being accurately and impartially? Not necessarily. At this point, our predicament should be no surprise since we still haven't established what someone's "core being" or "self" is. Without knowing exactly what we're searching for, we can't possibly know where to look, and even if by accident we happen to stumble across it, we won't be able to recognize what we see. Our situation, then, isn't so different from Peer Gynt's when he first set out to discover his elusive self.

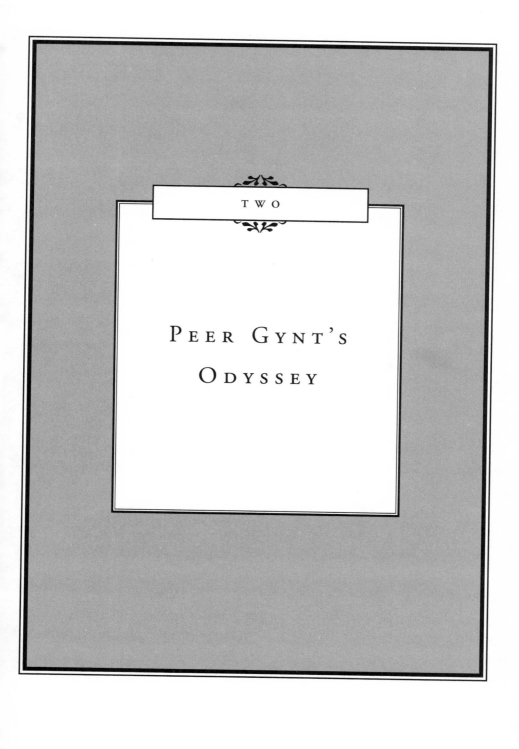

TWO

PEER GYNT'S ODYSSEY

SOME YEARS AGO, during my research on multiple personality, an incident made me realize just how naive my notions were about the self.[1] I concocted an informal experiment to help a person whom I was treating for multiple personality. The plan was to show Jonah, the primary personality, videotaped interviews of his three alter personalities, Usoffa Abdullah, King Young, and Sammy, all of whom were unknown to him. My intention was to get him to accept them as integral parts of himself. I assumed that once he saw himself in each of these different roles, he would immediately renounce his preposterous behaviors. I couldn't have been more wrong.

In the videotape, Usoffa Abdullah, son of Omega, who referred to himself as a god but not *the* God, and as the sworn defender of Jonah, glared at the camera and then at me, his interviewer, ready to strike out. Jonah, a pleasant, self-effacing black man of twenty-nine, watched the replay of this scene, unfazed by the belligerence of the stranger on the screen, who was his doppelgänger. The TV picture shifted to me, gently urging Usoffa to close his eyes and return to his hypnotic sleep. Grudgingly, he obliged. Then, after some coaxing on my part, King Young, known for his flirtatious behavior with women, opened his eyes, winked at me on screen, and grinned.

Jonah, still watching the film, showed no recognition of his alter personality.

After some conversation, I instructed King Young to close his eyes and go into a hypnotic sleep and then, after he did, I urged Sammy to come forth. Unlike Jonah, who was shy and inhibited, Sammy was a glib, lawyer type who prided himself on his rationality and spent much of his time getting Jonah out of the messes that Usoffa created.

Bored, Jonah shifted in his chair, paying little attention to the verbal shenanigans of his new alter ego on screen.

Then I asked Sammy to close his eyes and go into a deep hypnotic sleep, after which I instructed Jonah to come forth.

Now Jonah's attention was riveted to the screen. As the person on screen opened his eyes, Jonah shouted, "Hey, that's me!" Though he failed to recognize the alter personalities who inhabited the same body, Jonah immediately identified himself once his namesake emerged.

At first, Jonah's unanticipated response was puzzling. Yet later, the more I thought about it, the more sense it made. It was the only rational response to an irrational situation. How else should someone capable of these psychological gymnastics act? I already had established from my work with him that each of these personalities, although having access to the same fund of general information, such as where the interview was being held, how to spell or perform calculations, or who various people were, had specialized knowledge and memories in certain emotionally charged areas and had a distinctive demeanor. Just because these different entities inhabited the same body didn't necessarily give them the same identity.

No doubt, many people will be skeptical about the "genuineness" of Jonah's response because of the theatrics involved. But it isn't my purpose now to argue for the legitimacy of multiple personality. Nor do I want to explain how someone with a fragmented self can become a repository for a series of cardboard cutouts, living out their cartooned lives as if in rotogravure. I offer this anecdote to point out some of the complexities involved in an understanding of the self and to show that you can't always take the existence of a single, intact, personal self for granted.

Experiences of this sort needn't be pathological. I first became impressed with how a self can split some years ago in London when part of my own self took it upon itself to act contrary to my intentions. One day I decided to play hookey from a convention and wandered about in Soho, absorbing the sights. Soon I came upon a crowd of people on the sidewalk, gathered around a man deftly shifting three cards about on a small fold-up table and inviting bettors to guess which card was the ace. As I moved forward to gain a better view, a respectable-looking man next to the table snuck a peek under one card, which was clearly an ace, while the dealer was looking away, and then, when it came time for betting, asked me to put my hand over his chosen card as he reached for his money. He bet £25 and invited me to do the same as an apparent reward for my aid. I was suspicious that something was fishy even though I didn't know at the time that the man next to me was a shill. But my greed at winning this sure-fire bet got intense. I hesitated, wrestling with my decision. Maybe I should bet £50 since I saw with my own eyes that the down-turned card was the ace. Soon, the dealer became impatient with me and, abetted by the crowd, insisted that I quickly make up my mind. The more he pressured me, the more rattled I became. Then, finally, as I decided to make a bet, I reached with my left hand for my wallet. "My God! My wallet's gone," I gasped as I noticed my empty pocket. At this, the dealer folded the table, grabbed an aluminum case, and quickly disappeared. After the crowd evaporated and I began to walk away, puzzling whether it would do any good to report my missing wallet to the police, I was aware that I was not as upset as I should be, wandering about in a foreign city with my money and credit cards gone. Then the reason why became clear as I happened to look at my right hand. In it I held my wallet. No wonder I wasn't more distressed. In the moment of my being pressured to decide, some part of me acted to protect me from myself—keeping me from betting on something I sensed was a ruse—so that my avaricious left hand, literally, didn't know what my guardian right hand was doing.

The question is, who or what acted on my behalf? While grateful to whatever part of me had done so, I began to wonder what it meant. Was there some protective entity within me, a homunculus, an alter-personality of sorts, which could act independently of my conscious intentions, or was what happened irrelevant to my basic notion of self?[2]

While experiences like these are associated with amnesia and sometimes with dramatic acts, they aren't so different from those times during your life when you wonder what gets into you, what must have possessed you, when you seemingly act out of character: times when you say things you don't mean, when you do things you vow not to do, and when you act at odds with how you feel. It's perhaps at those times that you wish you had the capacity for dissociation, an exonerating amnesia that not only protects you from guilt but from the realization that you may not be in control of all you do.

In a sense, multiple personality has become a metaphor for our times. Once a rarity, it has become more commonplace, attesting not so much to the failure of clinicians to diagnose it in the past, but to a changing cultural climate that has allowed it and other disruptions in identity to flourish. Nowadays, as you explore the inner reaches of your mind, you stumble upon fragments of other selves, transitional figures, parental imagoes, guiding spirits, stunted and fixated selves from childhood, rudimentary beings, co-conscious entities, or nascent selves awaiting to emerge *de novo* under the right conditions, like Athena from the head of Zeus.[3] With the modern emphasis on synthetic identities, the human mind has become a foundry for new selves and a junkyard for discarded ones. Industries now exist that offer personality overhauls, attitude adjustments, packaged identities, and self-realization through seminars, workshops, courses, and self-help books. Cults or quasi-religious organizations have perfected techniques for reprogramming your mind. You're no longer bound to the constraints of your past. You now have the option to assume different persona or reinvent yourself.

THE CENTER OF AN ONION

How then do you go about discovering who you really are? This is Peer Gynt's dilemma in the play of the same name by Henrik Ibsen.[4] After a rambunctious and irresponsible youth, Gynt comes to see himself as a conglomerate of wishes, appetites, desires, ambitions, needs, and demands . . . "whatever causes my breast to heave uniquely, and makes me exist as the 'I' that I am." After traveling wide and far and adopting many identities, he compares his self to an onion that, after peeling each successive layer, is found to have no central core. Sometime later, when he confesses his unhappiness to a friend, his friend tells him that the only way for him to be himself is to obliterate his own identity through expressing the will of God. Unable to figure out what it is he should be expressing, Gynt eventually encounters a woman he deserted in his youth. She reveals to him that his true self has nothing to do with who he thinks he is, but that, despite the passage of years, it conforms to her loving remembrance of him. With that comforting news, he lays his head on her lap and finally allows himself to sleep.

What Ibsen portrays so well in his play isn't only the varying notions of the self—the self as a collection of drives and needs, and the self assuming different roles, each corresponding to the layers of an onion—but the different ways people view Gynt when he's in these roles. What Ibsen didn't say, but might have said if he added another act, was that Peer Gynt, after awakening from his newly beloved's lap, now becomes compelled to keep her from changing her loving image of him, because if she ever does change it, he'll have to begin his personal search anew.

Sometimes, as with Peer Gynt, people have to find their elusive self before they can know it. In her biography about Anne Sexton, Diane Middlebrook offers a portrait of a tormented poet who was so unsure about who she was that she sometimes doubted her own existence. "I am nothing, if not an actress off the stage," Sexton confesses. "It comes down to the terrible truth that there is no true part of me."[5]

Wary of Sexton's enigmatic pronouncements that there was no true part of her, I asked Middlebrook what she was trying to capture about her subject when she was trying to bring her to life.

"I was trying to capture her sense of a 'self.' It was a word she used a lot, and it was a word that had positive meanings for her. So not having one was a source of concern to her. Her associations with it chiefly had to do with her memory. When she would have memories that she couldn't trust, she doubted very much that she existed or had a self at all. The way this often expressed itself was when she told her therapist a story about an episode that she thought she remembered and then later doubted it. Sometimes she acknowledged awareness about telling a story that really wasn't true, but she associated that with her illness early on and later with her creativity. Gradually, she came to relinquish the idea that she needed to remember everything, because she saw that she could be a story teller without always being able to distinguish the truth. At one point, after working with her therapist for some time, she begins to tell him very excitedly she's discovered that poetry gives her a self for other people and therefore helps her to have one for herself. That was tremendously interesting to me because it wasn't as if there was something within her seeking expression. Her self was something that had to be located, an absent something that seemed elusive and troubling. It was established through the act of creativity that became her vocation."

What I interpreted Middlebrook to mean was that through the process of translating her perceptions and thoughts into poetry and realizing that she had something important to say, Sexton came to realize who she was. It became the *raison d'etre* for her existence. It was the emotional glue that held her together, even more than her family did. "You forced me to tell the truth," she wrote to one of her therapists, who rebuked her for putting her writing before her daughter. "The writing comes first. This is my way of mastering experience."[6] Yet, who is to say that Anne Sexton, the housewife and mother, is any less real than Anne Sexton, the poet, just because she believes herself to be and doesn't feel completely comfortable in these roles? Pursuing this issue, I asked Middlebrook if she believed there was such a thing as a real self versus a false self.

"It doesn't seem to me that you can distinguish the false from the true. The selves are pretty contextual."

"There are some people who might view the sense of self as a kind of fiction," I responded. "Do you?"

"Yes, definitely it's a fiction. The sense you have of yourself really is the result of having an unconscious and needing to control its access to the world, so to speak. But I also think that the way your behavior gets mirrored back to you gives you a lot of information that you use for your identity formation early in life. You have selves that are sort of localized within your career and life circumstances and the dynamics of relationships and all those things. When people act badly and don't know why, it shows what a thin and brittle construct the notion of the self is."

Though she didn't explicitly say so, Middlebrook seemed to be expressing one of the many paradoxes about the self. With little sense of a personal self beforehand, Anne Sexton presumably found her sense of self in her poetry, but the self she discovered may have had little to do with whom she "really" was. As I plan to show, this sense of self isn't necessarily equivalent to what a self is.

Yet for all of Peer Gynt's frustrations and failures, he knows that he exists and that there is an "I" hidden somewhere within, just as you know that you exist and have a self. This sense of self seems rooted in your being, not some abstruse concept, concocted by your consciousness, but intrinsic to every aspect of your existence, from the molecular to the social levels. Within your immune system, for instance, antibodies identify which molecules, cells, or tissues belong to you and which don't.[7] Those that are part of the non-self are attacked and destroyed. That's what happens when your body combats infection or rejects incompatible organ transplants. This molecular sense of self seems to become more defined over time. During infancy, when your immune system is immature and you're not yet able to identify yourself in the mirror, you borrow antibodies from your mother, a process known as passive immunity, until you become old enough to manufacture them yourself. With maturity, the immune system responds at two levels, one a nonspecific line of defense and the other an induced specific immunity. With the nonspecific line of defense, natural killer cells and macrophages respond quickly by attacking foreign bodies, such as tumor cells, bacteria, or viruses. When organisms get by this first line of defense, induced specific immune responses involving T-lymphocytes and B cells take over. This recognition of cells belonging to the self and those belonging to the non-self has survival value. It's when you don't have the capacity to destroy, eliminate, or neutralize foreign organisms or when your immune system fails to detect these potential threats that you're in mortal danger.

Unfortunately, the wisdom of your body is far from perfect. Certain forms of viruses or cancer cells seem to get by these natural lines of defense and expropriate the resources of your body as their own. Even more remarkable, with a variety of autoimmune diseases such as rheumatoid arthritis, polymyositis, lupus, myasthenia gravis, scleroderma, and certain thyroid disorders, the body either doesn't recognize certain of its own tissues as part of its self or misidentifies them as alien. As a result, it slowly destroys itself.

This confusion about what is part of the self and what isn't happens in other ways as well. Although the notion of your physical self covers almost anything within the boundaries of your body, including your hair, fingernails, urine, sputum, and feces, you're likely to become squeamish about these excrescences and disown them once they leave the sanctuary of your body.[8] In certain cultures, though, you may retain an irrational, primitive sense of possessiveness over your discarded bodily products, worried that your enemies may use them to make effigy dolls and cast spells over you.

Like a country's territorial waters, you also possess an invisible space outside of your skin, which defines your personal boundaries.[9] It sets the critical distance at which you feel comfortable relating to others in public and private encounters. When others intrusively enter this space without your invitation or approval, you feel vulnerable and instinctively prepare to retreat or attack. If this happens often enough, especially during your formative years when you're incapable of defending yourself, you may be forced, like a vanquished country, to surrender part of your personal territory, which, in turn, may contribute to a defective sense of self.

What all this points up is that your sense of self seems to pervade every level of your existence, from biochemical and cellular responses to psychological reactions and social behavior. It seems bred in your bones, a property of life itself. But as accurate as this sense of self may be, it isn't unerring. You know you exist, but not everything you identify as you is you and some of what you identify not as you may be.

You can note certain of these misperceptions in your sense of physical identity. Since childhood, for example, you've learned to identify yourself by the face you see staring back at you in the mirror. That's how you see yourself in your mind's eye and imagine how others see you and decide if you're worth knowing or not. Despite the identical correspondence of your mirror image with your physical body, many factors influence whether you subjectively identify your reflection as you. Brain damage to the non-dominant parietal lobe of your cerebral cortex from injury, tumor, or stroke may radically alter your body-image and keep you from recognizing one side of your face or body as belonging to you— a condition known as anosognosia. As a result, you may comb your hair only on one side of your head, shave or apply makeup only to one side of your face, or wash and dry only one side of your body. You even may believe that the extremities on one side of your body belong to somebody else.[10]

How then do you go about solving the mystery of a sense of self that is so intrinsic to your being, yet seems so malleable and elusive? Obviously, this is no easy task. But if you have any hope of ever doing so, you first need to know what the essential properties of the self are and also what they are not.[11]

IS CONDILLAC'S STATUE REAL?

In a little known work, *A Treatise on the Sensations*, published in 1754, the Abbé de Condillac, using a statue as a metaphor, argued that the progressive addition of the five senses gave rise to all higher mental faculties and formed the basis for the sense of self.[12] Needs arise when the statue remembers its past sensations, compares them to its present ones, and feels compelled to experience its former ones again. The statue gains its sense of "I-ness" by the simultaneous awareness of its current sensations and the memory of its prior ones.

While Condillac believed he was making a strong case for the five senses serving as the basis for the self, he was unintentionally making an even stronger one for the importance of memory. Once having gained the sense of smell, sight, hearing, taste, and touch, the statue's sense of "I-ness" could remain intact even if it systematically lost its senses one by one, as long as it remembered what it once sensed. This suggests that memory, or at least the intertwining of memory with sensations, may serve as a repository for the sense of self.

However, once you base your sense of self on memory, the very idea of a "self" becomes tenuous. At least, this is the argument of certain ultra-rationalist philosophers who use Descartes' famous dictum, "I think, therefore I am," as a convenient strawman for their discussions about the self. While Descartes' claim that you infer the existence of your self from your thought processes seems intuitively attractive—for who else could be thinking your thoughts except you?—others have argued that this doesn't represent *a priori* proof of the existence of a self. Your thoughts only prove the existence of a stream of consciousness. There is no logical basis to assume that this stream of consciousness belongs to some coherent, inner entity. John Locke and later David Hume, both early English philosophers, argued that since memory bridges the gaps in consciousness (and helps you to remember who you are each morning when you awaken), it alone underlies your sense of self. Hume reasoned that you have no actual experience of a self, no experience as an experiencer of your experiences. The self isn't a given. It is like a perceptual show taking place in a theater that doesn't exist.[13]

No doubt, despite these philosophical arguments, memory contributes significantly to your sense of self, but memory alone doesn't seem sufficient to explain it. If the sole basis for the self resides in memory, then people with Korsakoff's amnesia, severe Alzheimer's disease, or various dementias, who hardly can remember what has transpired from one moment to the next and often can't recall their own names or recognize their closest relatives, must have no sense of self even though they may be alert, respond to questions, and have moments of clarity. Yet this conclusion seems hard to justify when you find that many of these persons still enjoy certain creature comforts and sometimes even show glimmerings of an inner intelligence. Some argue that these individuals, as humans, retain their self until death, even though they lack the capacity to express it. The self presumably continues to exist in some coherent form within them, sometimes buried beneath psychological rubble or neural debris, much as it may during anesthesia or periods of unconsciousness. Whether this is true, naturally, depends on what you mean by a self.

CHINESE BOXES

What about the flip side of Descartes's dictum, which is, "I am, therefore I think," a position that equates the self with its products or functions, such as thinking, deciding, or behaving, and places its locus in consciousness. You are your acts, what you choose, says Søren Kierkegaard, an existentialist.[14] The only thing-in-itself that can't be thought is existence itself. The self unfolds when you identify with the results of your actions, says Hegel. The activity of the mind is the realization of itself. In dialectical fashion, the self as subject can also have itself as object. Though intriguing, these arguments ignore the fact that these products or functions don't necessarily prove the existence of the self. They don't adequately explain who or what chooses to act or decides to identify with certain acts. Logically, there also is no reason why "nonselves," such as computers or automata yet to be devised, shouldn't be capable of similar acts.

Immanuel Kant, the great German philosopher, tried to get around this problem by positing the existence of a *noumenal* self and a *phenomenal* self. The noumenal self is a self-in-itself, the "I am" that transcendentally accompanies every thought. A unified awareness of self and an awareness of the self as unified must exist before you can experience any later experience as yours. It is unknowable, operating outside the realm of causal order and, as such, can't be emulated by any rational or mechanical means, such as a computer. The necessity for a preexisting, knowing "I," as distinct from the observable actions of the self, haunts all later philosophical thought, from Schopenhaur to William James.[15]

In more recent times, Julian Jaynes transforms the self as knower into the self as narrator.[16] He argues that your sense of personal consciousness couldn't have arisen without the development of written language. Written language, representing a document of what transpired before, liberates you from the dominating influence of your right brain and the commanding, hallucinatory voices that often arise from it during dreamy states and that you're likely to ascribe to supernatural agencies. Once you can place the emotional impact of a moment within a written, historical context, to be contemplated rather than acted upon immediately, you become able to act on your own initiative and regulate your own life. You now can conceive of a "self," an analog "I," that can move about vicariously in your imagination, doing things that you actually aren't doing, or of a metaphor "me" that can look out from within your imagined self at the imagined people and the imagined scenes. This "self" exists in consciousness, makes choices, and acts as in a story.

So far in my selective review, I've described theories about the self that base its existence on the sensations, on memory, and on consciousness. Then within consciousness I've identified an observer, a narrator, or an executor self that functions as the "I" (the self as subject), and an observed self that functions as the "me" (the self as object) and has attributes that it identifies as "mine." The "I," as with Kant's noumenal self, is devoid of human qualities, a mostly dispassionate and sometimes judgmental observer of the all-too-human observed self, the "me." It is a beam of concerned awareness constantly directed toward the mental, emotional, and behavioral activities of the observed self, which usually are associated with personal identity.

Unfortunately, what should clarify the nature of the self only confounds it more, since now you have a conceptual dilemma, reminiscent of that posed by Heisenberg's indeterminacy principle for quantum physics, which is that the measuring process itself alters what it's measuring. Whenever you observe a phenomenon in Nature, especially at the atomic level, you don't observe this phenomenon itself but only the phenomenon exposed to the nature of your observations. With different forms of observation, you should observe the phenomenon differently. When you apply this principle to the interplay between an observer self and an observed self, you find that whenever the observer within you directs its focus on the observable aspects of your self, the object of its observations becomes immobilized, much like a deer transfixed by the glow of powerful headlights. For instance, when persons become self-conscious about their sexual responses with their partners, a condition known as "spectatoring," their natural responsiveness becomes impaired. Paradoxically, the observer self can only capture the natural activity of the observed self when it's not actively observing it.

Aside from the distorting effects of the observer on the observed event, suggesting that you never can be an objective observer of yourself, the major problem with theories about the self that conceive of a preexisting, unknowable something—Plato's charioteer, representing reason, who drives the twin steeds of appetite and ambition; Kant's transcendental self-in-itself; William James's pure ego; or a host of other metaphors used to characterize the unfathomable—is that they explain nothing at all. Now, instead of the mind as the source of self-directed thought and activity, you have an elfin homunculus within it, adorned in various conceptual attire, a genie of sorts, as the real overseer of your thoughts, feelings, and behaviors. The problem with all of these metaphors is that they inevitably lead you into a logical trap. Once you propose the existence of an executive ego, the self becomes a Chinese box in which the larger box has a smaller box within it, and the smaller box has an even smaller box, since you now have to propose the existence of a sub-homunculus directing the homunculus, and so on, *ad absurdum*. Faced with this dilemma, most self-respecting theories about the self arbitrarily adopt a Trumanesque, the-buck-stops-here stance for the proposed *a priori* observer self, making it an originator or irreducible given. The homunculus becomes self-causing. However, once the observer self acquires this divine-like status, you're obliged to echo the philosopher's response to the claim that God created the universe: "But who created God?"

CAN FALSE SELVES BE TRUE?

With the advent of psychoanalysis, other puzzles about the self emerge. Now you find that even the self that is capable of being observed and studied mostly remains unknown. Like the tip of an iceberg, it's only partly revealed, not only because of the instinctual forces acting upon it, but because it uses numerous defense mechanisms to deceive itself, mainly to keep you from experiencing anxiety. The Freudian self is tripartite, consisting of an executive *ego* that constantly mediates between an instinctual *id* that houses unconscious wishes, and a *super-ego* that exerts social prohibitions and expectations. Though couched in more mystical language, Carl Jung's self has most of the same characteristics. It represents a master archetype for organizing experience. It includes a *persona*, representing the public mask and the conventional roles people adopt, and the *shadow*, which is the repository for all instinctual, biological forces.

Implicit in these views are three overlapping but somewhat different portrayals of the self: the false versus the true self, the known versus the unknown self, and the private versus the public self.[17] Supposedly, the false self is inhibited and guilt-ridden, characterized by artificiality and self-deception, whereas the true self is spontaneous, guilt-free, and genuine, unfettered by any emotional impediments. The known self is that part of you accessible to consciousness and reflection, while the unknown self resides in your unconscious, dominated largely by subterranean, instinctual forces and best revealed through dreams and fantasies. The private self includes all of your thoughts, feelings, and actions that aren't observable by others, while the public self involves those aspects of yourself that are open to public scrutiny.

While clinically useful, these distinctions create conceptual nightmares. Why is a conflicted and inhibited self any less "true" than a nonconflicted and spontaneous one? This artificial distinction seems to have contributed to Anne Sexton's confusion about the reality of her self. Each self is as real to the person experiencing it and as much the product of natural forces as the other. All that the distinction between a true and a false self signifies is a value judgment, and a not necessarily defensible one at that, which arbitrarily presupposes that the absence of all conflict represents the most natural state.

Why is your private self a truer reflection of your real self than the self you expose to the public? Because you have fantasies, motives, and aspirations that are secret doesn't mean that they aren't as much shaped by psychological conflicts and social expectations and potentially as misrepresentative of your natural inclinations as your public behaviors may be.

Yet another issue has to do with the notion of the self as partly known but mostly unknown, with the known part mostly composed of all the rationalizations, distortions, and falsifications you unknowingly use to protect yourself from guilt and to justify what you say and do—a self largely contaminated by self-serving error. This implies that you may not be the person you believe yourself to be since you remain ignorant of all the unconscious forces that control you.

The idea that you possess a self that employs defense mechanisms to shield you from information that may be emotionally unsettling is mind-boggling. Just think what it means to have a self that engages in self-deception.[18] It means that the self, much as a concerned parent, has the capacity to protect the vulnerable aspects of itself from disturbing knowledge by hiding certain information from itself, censoring it, or modifying it to make it more palatable. To deceive itself, the self must simultaneously believe what it knows to be false and deny what it knows to be true, acting much like an alcoholic who hides a bottle of liquor from himself to keep from drinking but always knowing where it's hidden. As preposterous as this seems, something of this sort seems to be happening with multiple personalities.

"In terms of this issue of capturing a person," I asked Victor Bockris, the noted biographer and friend of Andy Warhol, as well as the author of books about Keith Richards and William Burroughs, "do you believe that there is such as a thing as a self? You know there is a lot of philosophical speculation about whether it exists? Do people create it? How much do people invent themselves?"

"There is a self only in as much as you believe there is a self. Basically we hold ourselves together day by day by not dwelling on it but by having some image of ourselves. We create our own images. I'm a certain age, living in a certain area, involved in a certain type of career, which creates an image of me, which is basically what I want to be. I am doing what I want to do and being what I want to be, so that's me. I'm also aware that I have at least two or three very changeable personalities. I'm not schizophrenic in the sense of my behavior to other people, but internally I'm aware of being able to visit or be visited by different aspects of myself, which I recognize as some of my hangovers from childhood. Some of them are partially self-created fantasy characters based upon performances and from habit over the years.

"These are not radical things. To me, it's almost like connections to other intelligences in yourself, other than the state you portray to the world. I like to operate on more than that. That state, to some extent, is an act. Andy used to say that he put on his Andy Warhol suit every morning when he got up. Andy lived as if his whole life was a movie in which he was starring, and he actually put on a costume and makeup in the morning before he went out. Once he hit the street, he was on, he was Andy Warhol, literally. He was acting in the street. He used to give magazines away and give autographs in the street. He liked it. It was part of the whole aura of being this famous celebrity in New York.

"To some extent we all do that, particularly people who go to an office everyday and have to dress and act in a certain way and obey orders. Obviously, they're acting more than those of us who have the luxury of working in our own offices. But we all have to conform. We are all created largely by the law, custom, and society. We pretty much sleep at the same time, eat at the same time, and do all the same things. We put that together with our own act, and we've got a lot to juggle. Just to keep all that going is a full-time job.

"That's why I like to be able to have connections with other intelligences. These are the intelligence connections through dreams, through art, and particularly for me, through writing and reading. I'm a person who spends a lot of time alone writing, so that I have a lot of conversations with myself and with other people constantly . . . my characters, obviously, and people I know. So all those things are operating."

CAN SELVES ACTUALIZE THEMSELVES?

How stable is the self? Are you accorded one self that remains relatively the same throughout the life cycle or does it change as you develop and mature? Is it your task to discover and express that true, inner self or to nurture an incomplete, immature self so that, as the popular saying goes, it eventually can be all that it can be? As it happens, the notion of a stable self, which some equate with the mind, awareness, consciousness, or even the soul, presents conceptual problems. If the contents of the mind change, David Hume would argue, then the self, which is dependent upon the mind, must too. But the notion of a changing, evolving self also has its theoretical pitfalls.

While the notion of a substantial, enduring self that remains the same through infancy, childhood, adulthood, and old age seems difficult to fathom, it's well suited to the belief in an immortal soul, one immune to the ravages of time and the travails you experience in life. It is the enduring part of you, which is in potential touch with the eternal. It is imprisoned in your body, which serves as a temporary caretaker or waystation for this precious entity that, according to certain beliefs, can be saved if lost or become reunited with God or stand in your stead as a spectral defendant when your accumulated sins and good deeds are scrutinized on Judgement Day. As appealing as the belief in an irreducible, immaterial, shadowy, eternal representation of you may be, it wreaks havoc with any rational understanding of the self. Even Peer Gynt, who temporarily embraced the idea of the self as soul, had trouble figuring out how a self could be selfless while at the same time expressing divine intention.

According to the philosopher A. N. Whitehead, there is no same self since it's always in flux.[19] It represents a composite at any given time of an evolving series of creative moments, an organizational unity of those that are contemporaneous and those that are successive. It comes into being by incorporating what is perishing with what is transpiring in the present. As such, the self is the same yet different, a process rather than an entity. Other writers, such as Abraham Maslow or Eric Erickson, emphasize the changing nature of personal identity over a succession of life stages or the striving for self-realization through the processes of self-actualization. These notions are all based on the assumption that you need to remove the impediments to self-knowledge to experience the progressive unfolding of your self and become who you are meant to be.[20]

What is especially troubling about most notions of an actualized self is the unspoken, elitist assumption that people are somehow deficient in selfhood if they fail to achieve this psychological state of grace. Achieving this ideal of self-actualization isn't something that happens automatically to everyone, like physical maturity, but occurs only in the enlightened few who find ways to overcome the impediments. But arguments for why an actualized self rather than one encrusted with traditional beliefs or plagued by conflicts should be a truer expression of your self aren't convincing. More to the point, it's difficult to understand the nature of a self that can launch a search party to discover the hidden, yet unrealized dimensions of itself and that keeps changing with each clue it uncovers. Then, when it presumably arrives at its unknown destination, which lacks identifiable signposts, how can it ever be sure it's where it set out to be?

> "It seems perhaps more than anyone I've read that this issue of identity was so important to Virginia Woolf," I commented to Louise DeSalvo, her biographer. "For example, in *Orlando*, she made all of the comments

about the fluidity of the self, the multiple selves, things along these lines. Do you also see her as trying to make sense out of who she was?"

"I see her as being extremely involved in understanding this issue, perhaps further along than people writing in other fields were. I see her as understanding the fundamental issue that the self is in flux, and that any time we begin to study who we are, the self becomes an elusive entity. Because even as we're trying to figure out who we are now, we are in the process of changing in an ongoing dialectic with the people around us in the world. So the very attempt to do this has to be understood as being a tentative attempt, because we can never grasp the cardinal issue of who we are. It's very Eastern in its own way, very non-Western . . . a kind of fundamental understanding that the self is in flux, that there is no such stable entity through time, but that nonetheless there is a kind of cosmic center within that is whole and that has to be trusted. So I do see her as dealing with the notion of the fluidity of the self, . . . the very garments we put on in order to conduct our lives with various people so that we appear in one way to one person and another way to another person."

A "ME" SELF OR A "WE" SELF?

Another important issue about the nature of the self has to do with whether it represents an autonomous entity that operates independently of others or whether it exists only as a part of a social system. Supposedly, an autonomous self, with its emphasis on the "me," is an island unto itself that remains intact and coherent despite the many forces acting upon it. Its orientation is toward the fulfillment of its own intentions and needs. It is, so to speak, the master of its fate and the captain of its soul. This emphasis on an autonomous "me," as distinct from the selves of others, is more prevalent in Western cultures, particularly America, than non-Western cultures. It is a self that embodies both the positive qualities of self-sufficiency and independence, and the negative qualities of selfishness and egocentricity. In contrast, the "we" self, with its focus on other people, represents the product of social interactions. In non-Western cultures, such as Asia, Africa, parts of the Middle East and Indonesia, for example, or in certain Western subcultures, such as the Amish, the emphasis is primarily on the family, group, or society. People are part of a larger social network, gaining their personal identity from their connectedness with others. Unlike the independent "me" self, whose goal is to express itself, the interdependent "we" self works at being attuned to what others are thinking and feeling and at responding to their particular needs.[21]

As may be expected, the relative extent of me-ness or we-ness within a culture or subculture seems to have a profound effect on its customs and values. The greater the culture's reverence for the self, the greater its respect for privacy, personal space, and personhood, and the more likely it will foster more personalized forms of improvisation and creative expression, such as autobiographies, individual musical performances, confessional poetry, or idiosyncratic forms of art. The greater the premium it places on kinship and work groups, the less its emphasis on privacy, personal space, and personhood, and the greater its emphasis on anonymity, tradition, and less personal forms of creative expression.[22]

Near the turn of the century, C. F. Cooley coined the term, the *looking glass self,* to account for the many ways that social interactions influence the sense of self and shape human behavior. In effect, he claimed that you see yourself mainly through the eyes of others or how you imagine their responses to you, and form your opinions about yourself from these real and imagined responses. Later, George Herbert Meade, a social psychologist, adopted a similar approach, explaining the self's unique capacity to reflect on itself as a function of social interaction and the acquisition of language.[23]

Though the emphasis on the "me" or the "we" undoubtedly contributes to your self-concept, either emphasis alone seems deficient. A self that is completely independent of other selves or cultural influences is a preposterous notion since it ignores the reality of all the psychological and social programming that you are exposed to and that shapes your attitudes and actions. Also, the notion of an autonomous self, carried to an extreme, isn't too far removed from the position of solipsism, whereby a completely self-contained mind not only creates its own reality but also imagines the existence of other selves.

While social psychological theories offer an important perspective on the nature of the self, especially explaining how you can be "different" people in different social settings, they also have serious limitations. Not only do they fail to account for the source and nature of your *"I"* that imagines what others think of it and manages to selectively expropriate others' attitudes as your own, but they also ignore the implications of your own attempts to manipulate the opinions of others so that they think well of you. Undoubtedly, early in your life, the attitudes of your parents and other important authority figures toward you have a profound effect on how you see yourself, but as time goes by, you increasingly seek to influence how others respond to you. In essence, then, you have a situation whereby you try to shape the opinions of others in a certain fashion so that they conform to the opinions you want them to have about you or you already have about yourself.

DECONSTRUCTING THE SELF

What can you conclude so far from this brief review of theories about the self? One important observation is that no single theory seems to capture adequately all the dimensions of the self. Another is that if you grant at least some credence to each of the main theories, the self appears to represent an elastic construct with mutually contradictory properties. It is part true and part false. It is part known and part unknown. It is part public and part private. It simultaneously preexists and is in the process of coming into being. It is part observing and part observed. And it is both independent and interdependent, part "me" and part "we."

To complicate matters, notions about the self also seem to be influenced by historical and social forces. These changing notions tend to be reflected in representative biographical accounts of the times.[24] For instance, James Boswell's exhaustive, eighteenth-century biography of Samuel Johnson, which serves as a landmark in the depiction of character, suggested that the proper study of people dealt with everything they did, said, or thought. Even their bills, appointment schedules, or mannerisms revealed important dimensions about their characters. This biographical account likely influenced William James's view that the self was the sum of everything you accepted as belonging to you, including your body, possessions, social role, feelings, and values. It certainly seemed to serve as a model for Leon Edel's own monumental work.

Leon Edel was one of the first modern biographers to explain how the biographer, as a participant-observer, creatively imposed a narrative structure on his subject's life. His classic, five-volume biography of Henry James, which took him more than twenty years to write and rivals Boswell's biography of Samuel Johnson, continues to serve as a model for thoroughness, in-depth understanding about the character of a person, and the imaginative structuring of facts. The biographer may be as imaginative as he pleases—the more imaginative the better—in the way he brings together his materials, says Edel, *but he must not imagine the materials.* Because his distinction between the biographical and fictional approach to the construction of persons has had a profound impact on modern theories about biography, his comments to me set the stage for certain of my later comments about the biographical nature of the self.

"How do you see your role as different from that of a novelist who is writing about a character?" I asked.

"The difference is," he answered, "I'm using one kind of imagination and a novelist uses a different kind. The novelist is omniscient. He or she can follow their imagination. They are fictionalizing. The novelist is going through a very complicated process of fictionalizing emotions and experiences to tell a story. I, as a literary biographer, which is my specialty, write books about actual, not fictional, people who were or are my subjects. I would, in these circumstances, have to look for each kind of life's myth and story that emerges from the data, the documentation. I read the writings of novelists, and what they have imagined . . . their fantasies of creation: these provide clues, patterns, life-views, and a philosophy of life."

"So in the construction of the character that you're writing about, you feel you are using a good deal of imagination in . . ." I began this loaded question, hoping that he would confirm my notion that these imaginative processes are not so different for biographers and novelists, but he didn't bite.

"No, my imagination is used in finding a structure and form. The biographer can be imaginative but mustn't imagine the facts. An archive usually contains thousands of letters and thousands of other documents, and you can't throw these at a reader. You can't even condense them, and there's no point in trying to do so. You extract *essence.* You constantly summarize conclusions drawn from your data. You describe what the documents have to reveal to you. . . . You become intuitive. You use inference. You speculate. You develop a hypothesis. You test one bit of evidence against another. That's the way a scientist works."

I wasn't convinced. How, I wondered, can biographers objectively construct a character from the myriad of self-serving fictions and biased interpretations contained within the materials they work with—autobiographical accounts, letters, memoirs—often written by their subjects to put themselves in the best light? But I already suspected how he might have answered. The task of the biographer is to detect the patterns and modes of a person's works and productions, or, to use Edel's own analogy, *the figure on the underside of the carpet*. Only by grasping the private mythology hidden behind the person's public mask can you depict the real person.

Perhaps as a natural elaboration of Boswell's approach, which suggested that a person was everything that you could learn about him, Lytton Strachey sought to illuminate the hidden self. Borrowing insights from Freud's writings, he used a psychobiographical approach in his *Eminent Victorians* to portray the double lives of his subjects, describing what went on in their minds and how their public behaviors and private motives often were at odds. Beneath the solid surface of behavior was an unseen, nebulous world of thought and fantasy.

In his accounts of Leonardo da Vinci and Moses and his detailed case studies, Sigmund Freud, in the early part of this century, consolidated the shift to the inner motives and often unconscious psychological processes of people. By placing people under the psychological microscope, biographers seemingly now had a way to identify the hidden motivations of their subjects.

Perhaps inspired partly by the writings of Marcel Proust and James Joyce, Virginia Woolf was likely the first biographer to deconstruct conventional notions of the self by depicting the fictional and illusory nature of personal identity. Rebelling against the traditional formulas used by her father, Leslie Stephen, the respected editor of the monumental *Dictionary of National Biography*, Woolf published *Orlando*, a pseudo-biographical account of a character who lived in several centuries and changed from a man to woman, and then *Flush*, an imaginative biography of a red cocker spaniel. What is so remarkable about *Orlando*, which supposedly was based on the life of her friend Vita Sackville-West, but which I suspect also reflected her own struggles with her personal identity, are her observations about the fluidity and multiplicity of the self. "Biography is considered complete," she astutely observed, "if it merely accounts for six or seven selves, whereas a person may well have as many as a thousand."[25]

I asked Louise DeSalvo, later in our interview, what she thought about my observation that Virginia Woolf was probably rebelling against her father after his death by abandoning many of the conventional laws of biography. "She took everything he stood for and systematically tore it apart," I commented.

"In the context of current literary critical theory, she deconstructed biography, whereas her father constructed biography . . . ," she answered. "I would say that she's trying to extend her father's notion of what the self is. In addition to fracturing his notion of how a life should be written, she's also fracturing his sense of what the self is . . . a stable entity through time who is judged on the basis of her or his accomplishments . . . marital status, and all that. I think she's doing a much fuller exploration of self."

In Norman Mailer's biography of Marilyn Monroe, in which he tried to fit his image of her to the imagined facts, and in his later book, which describes imaginary interviews with her, we take another step toward deconstructing conventional notions of the self.[26] Who someone is not only depends now on the biased perceptions of the perceiver but on "facts" that are contaminated by fiction and invented for the media. These "factoids" assume the mantle of truth, as people come to construct their lives around them. Because they no longer are bound by objective data, they now acquire the ability to invent themselves by creating identities of their own choosing.

PUTTING HUMPTY DUMPTY TOGETHER

These modern notions of the self add a new wrinkle to Descartes's dictum, which now becomes "I think I am, therefore I am." Perhaps the most dramatic example of a deconstructed self is a multiple personality, in whom fragments of persons, partial identities, emotional specialists, quasi-individuals, and two-dimensional entities inhabit the same body and appear and disappear at will, usually leaving the primary personality ineffectual and emotionally drained. This decomposition of the self is of more than theoretical interest. It poses mind-boggling, practical problems for a therapist, whose challenge, so to speak, is how to put Humpty Dumpty back together again.

With the treatment of my own patient, Jonah, for instance, I faced a number of personal and clinical dilemmas. The first dilemma was how seriously to take what I was doing. No matter how much objective evidence I gathered to show that each of the quasi-personalities led a relatively independent psychological existence, whenever I put him under hypnosis to call forth his alter egos, I had to keep fighting my feeling that he and I were locked in a *folie-à-deux*. Still, the mind works in strange ways, I constantly reminded myself, and if I wanted to maintain my patient's trust, I had to treat him and his entourage with respect.

Once having resolved to take the existence of these disparate personalities seriously, the next dilemma I faced was what to do with them. Although different clinicians advocate different treatment approaches, no scientific evidence existed to show that any given approach was substantially better than another. Should I work exclusively with Jonah, much as I do with patients with repressed, painful memories, to try to make him more aware of the hidden feelings that his alter selves represented? But then, I already found him singularly uninterested in these other inhabitants of his mind and doubted that he'd be motivated to pursue this. Should I treat each of the four entities separately with the goal of resolving the conflicts of each and affecting a reconciliation among them? But from my existing contacts with these entities, I already knew what to expect. Jonah would do whatever I asked him to, Usoffa would be uncooperative, Sammy would try any reasonable approach, and King Young would be too happy-go-lucky to change. Or should I work with one particular personality with the intention of making him dominant over all the others?

My initial inclination was to adopt this last option. Jonah, the primary personality, would be the logical selection, but he was too inept and passive to handle all the unruly personalities within him. Usoffa was out because he was too nasty. My preference was to promote Sammy to prominence because of his analytic reasoning and potential lawyerly ability to represent all elements of Jonah effectively. A colleague's choice was King Young because of his glibness and charm. Unable to settle on a particular personality, I decided to abandon this discriminatory approach in favor of complete integration, reasoning that it was better for all parties to be united than not. After all, I told myself, selves are supposed to be whole, or at least, that's what common lore holds,.

My plan was easier to devise than implement. During extensive negotiations with these personalities, whom I called forth separately under hypnosis, I tried to convince each that his individual interests could be better served if he became fused with the others and that continuation of this laissez faire arrangement could only lead to disaster for all. Unfortunately, my shuttle diplomacy of negotiating with one personality and then the next broke down, mainly because none of the other personalities wanted to forfeit his individual autonomy.

It was weeks later that the conceptual breakthrough occurred. I shared my inspiration with Jonah, Usoffa, Sammy, and King Young separately, and after some reluctance on their parts, each accepted my terms. By agreeing to become a confederation, they each could have equal representation in a new personality, JUSKY, an appellation that combined the first letters of each of their names. Don't laugh. It worked. This uneasy alliance of personalities continued for years, without any major internecine warfare and with only an occasional squabble.

Aside from certain quirks of mine, what this case of multiple personality shows is how fluid and fickle the nature of personal identity sometimes can be. Under exceptional circumstances, seemingly new beings can emerge, not necessarily from whole cloth but from the personal material already on hand. Though artificial, these beings aren't necessarily unreal. They can have agendas of their own, serve important emotional purposes, and function adequately in society. They also raise important questions about the nature of the self and the formation of personal identity. For example, just who is JUSKY, né Jonah? Does he qualify as a person? Does he have a real self? Most important, in what essential ways, if any, is he substantially different from people who lead double lives or hide behind a public persona or disguise perceived social flaws? What the discussion so far suggests is that there is much about current notions of the self that seems to border on science fiction and that people don't have to be multiple personalities to lead make-believe lives.

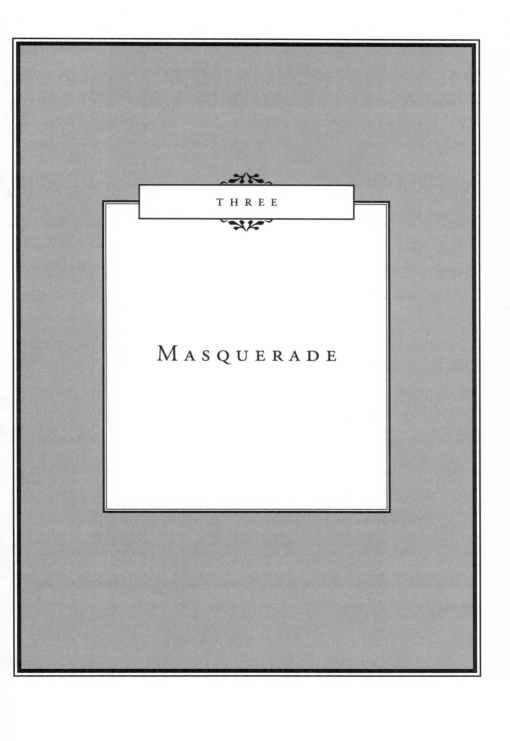

THREE

MASQUERADE

I N MY CONVERSATION WITH ARNOLD RAMPERSAD, a professor of English at Princeton University and the noted biographer of several eminent African Americans, I mentioned my view that much of our personal sense of identity is artificial because of its contextual, historical, and social basis. He readily agreed, and then added, "I have a friend who has been working on a big study about blacks in the schools and talking about plagiarized identities, which is a term that sets my teeth on edge. She talks about these blacks not performing well and hating school because they resent people who have plagiarized identities. My response has been for a long time that all identity is plagiarized. It's all copied. So where is the self . . . ?"

No doubt that a good part of your personal identity is knowingly or unknowingly "borrowed" from others. You model yourself after your mother or father, an older sibling, a favorite relative, a teacher, a mentor, a well-known athlete, a movie star, or a celebrity. You adopt the attitudes of people in your church, organization, group, team, or gang. Even when you rebel against your background or teachings, you're likely to assume another standardized, preformed identity, already packaged for unconventional and nonconforming types. This issue of personal identity creates a particular dilemma for African Americans who wish to succeed in a predominantly white culture yet seek their own distinctive identity. Whatever course they take, they must adopt identities that have a seal of approval either for whites or for blacks. This puts them in a no-win situation. They never can be "white" enough to be fully accepted by whites, and simply by virtue of adopting white standards for success, they never can be "black" enough for many blacks.[1]

In his now classical book, *Invisible Man*, Ralph Ellison articulates this dilemma well. In the opening pages, his nameless protagonist proclaims that he is "invisible" because people refuse to see him, and that when they approach him, they see only his surroundings, themselves, or figments of their imagination— everything and anything except him. Searching for his own identity, much as Peer Gynt tried to find his self, he first went to college to become better educated. After being expelled, he found acceptance by becoming active in the Brotherhood. Eventually, he became disillusioned with that, too, and retreated underground to the darkness of a manhole. There, in his isolation, he could avoid the absurdity of identity in America and contemplate in peace, concluding, "one of the greatest jokes in the world is the spectacle of whites busy escaping blackness and becoming blacker every day, and the blacks striving toward whiteness, becoming quite dull and gray. None of us seems to know who he is or where he's going."[2]

This feeling of being invisible extends beyond race. It can apply to any people who feel negatively typecast by others on the basis of what they perceive to be unjust, arbitrary, or artificial standards that potentially place them at a social disadvantage. Along with the anger toward an imperceptive society that feeling "invisible" can generate, it may affect their entire sense of self. It not only heightens confusion about who they are but may make the issue of their personal identity the *raison d'etre* of their existence. This prompts them to adopt some form of social camouflage, which either hides or accentuates their presumed differentness.

CROSSING THE LINE

I have a friend, I'll call him "Maxwell Wolffe," whom everybody admires and respects. He is handsome and charming. He is kindly and wise. He is a distinguished, corporate lawyer. He is a deacon in his church and a leader in the community. He is what everybody aspires to, the embodiment of respectability and success and integrity. He is a "Christian" in the best sense of the word. And yet, though he seems emotionally stable and contented, I begin to detect after long acquaintance a compulsiveness behind his solicitude, an edge of cynicism to his remarks, and an evasiveness to inquiries about his past, which makes me wonder, Is Max who he appears to be?

One evening, on a walk after dinner, Max tells me about a dream he has had. He tries to make light of it, but I can tell he is disturbed. For years, he reveals, he has been suffering from recurrent nightmares, with always the same theme and always the same sickening feeling after awakening, lingering well into the day, that what he dreams may be real. In the dream, he senses that he has committed some terrible crime long ago, presumably a murder, with the corpse or evidence buried in the basement of his house. The police or authorities are about to begin digging. Certain of imminent discovery, he's overwhelmed by apprehension as he anticipates the ruination of his career and the shock of all those who know him. Much like Joseph K., the respectable bank functionary in *The Trial*, and probably for the same reason that drove Franz Kafka to write so eloquently about irrational guilt and social alienation, he prepares to defend himself against an unspecified charge. He knows he's guilty but he's not sure of what. But as Max and I talk about the dream, his face suddenly blanches as its meaning becomes clear. I ask him what is wrong. He hesitates, then unexpectedly confesses to me, "I know now what the unmentionable crime is. I was born a Jew."

I introduce my friend to you to raise certain issues that apply to everyone seeking social acceptance, the foremost of which is "Who is he?" Is he the person almost all people think they know, or the person hardly anyone knows fully, not even his children and wife? Is his life built on a solid foundation of good deeds and honest interactions, or is it predicated on deceit and fiction? Or does it really matter?

Not all people who potentially are able to pass in society try to disguise their pasts. Some trumpet their pasts. But in their need to divulge their social flaw, they paradoxically may be announcing who they are not. Take Kirk Douglas, the actor, for instance. Born Issur Danielovitch Demsky, the son of an illiterate, immigrant, Russian-Jewish ragman, he describes in his best-selling autobiography his shame over his background—his father's occupation, his poverty, his Jewishness—and the lifelong anger this fuels.[3] His later accomplishments do little to stifle the hated, mocking Issur who always lurks in the background, reminding him of his humble and embarrassing origins and the ephemeral nature of his success. But does this open acknowledgment of these two selves within him make Douglas, now in his seventies, any more "real" than my friend? Though Douglas keeps professing his Jewishness, sometimes tauntingly so, you wonder about the legitimacy of his claim, considering his adopted WASPish name, his rugged, Aryan looks, his two marriages, each time to a "shiksa," his deliberate decision to allow his four sons to choose their own religion, if any, and only going to synagogue once a year, on Yom Kippur. What is it then that makes him "Jewish"? And do frank confessionals of this sort make him authentic or only reflect how authentic people are supposed to act?

The ways my friend and Kirk Douglas handle their supposed Jewishness, one escaping from it and the other proclaiming it, aren't so different from how most people in a position to "pass" in society or gain social acceptance handle the ambiguous, defining qualities about themselves (such as their religious backgrounds, ethnic origins, skin color, education, physical appearance, emotional difficulties, intelligence, social class, or sexual orientation), which potentially put them at a social disadvantage. Often, these presumed "flaws" can become the center of their personal existence and influence how they see themselves. This is especially so when they happen to be cast in the role of social pariah by birth or circumstance.

Take "Randall Marlow," for instance. Though recovering from a stroke, which left him partially paralyzed and with some difficulty in speaking, he displays a keen curiosity about almost everything and a sparkling but at times mordant wit. An acclaimed mathematician who holds a tenured professorship at an Ivy League university, he has every reason to feel proud of his accomplishments as he approaches retirement. He has attended the finest schools, has garnered many scientific honors, and has produced a number of highly touted if not classic works. A confirmed bachelor, he has numerous friends, and never seems to lack for something to do. Yet for all his social popularity and outward professional success, he is miserable, forever struggling against the beckoning embrace of suicide, and hardly anyone knows about it. The reason that none of his accomplishments matter is that he believes himself a fraud. He is a homosexual. He is ashamed of his humble origins. He distrusts his intelligence. And he has spent a good part of his life cultivating a façade to keep people from knowing.

With such an outlook, a constant fear of public exposure, naturally, colors all of Professor Marlow's life. Though hungering for intimacy and affection, he avoids gay hangouts, even when out of town, for fear of being identified for what he is. He avoids speaking out on controversial issues for fear that someone he offends may retaliate by taking it upon himself to investigate his life. He shuns close friendships with attractive men for fear that they will be able to read his mind or he will not be able to control his feelings. He derogates his own kindnesses to others because of his self-interest in wanting to be liked. He devalues his professional research and writings as either being unoriginal or not as worthy as those of others. And, when he really gets disgusted with himself, he regards his entire life a sham and himself a coward for not being courageous enough to speak out and not care what others think.

Whenever I think about Professor Marlow's plight, I become saddened. What a shame that someone with his many gifts and achievements does not feel better about himself! What a waste for him to base his opinion about himself and the worthwhileness of his life on his sexual orientation alone. Yet I realize that his response isn't uncommon for someone brought up to believe that homosexuality is an abomination and something to be ashamed of. Even Leonard Bernstein, who had countless, devoted fans and whose professional position was secure, by certain accounts, could see his whole life as a fraud because of his hidden stigma.

Humphrey Burton, now artistic advisor to the Barbican Centre in London and a longtime friend and director of film and television for Leonard Bernstein, as well as his biographer, said that Bernstein, in his later years, believed that he had lived a lie and falsified his life because he was more homosexual than heterosexual.

I asked Burton whether Bernstein had a firm sense of who he was.

"I think he had a very great sense of who he was, partly because of his extreme awareness of every aspect of the world going on around him and partly because he had from an early age consorted with various analysts and spent a lot of time talking about himself. I think he also knew that he was a very complex and multifaceted personality who had many different personalities, all jostling for position within him.

"When he was quite young, he told his girlfriends that he felt himself to have a chancre in his soul. There was a dark side to himself, he said at one time, which was probably a reference to his homosexuality. But he also wished to be thought of as a good, upright, heterosexual young man who was on the lookout for a wife. So there was this division within himself."

When you believe you have something to hide, as my friend Maxwell Wolffe and Professor Marlow believe they do, then your options for openness and self-expression become markedly reduced.[4] What happens is that you begin restricting or manipulating or manufacturing information about yourself in order to promote an acceptable public image or prevent an unacceptable one from being uncovered. One of the best ways to do this is by avoidance. You avoid encounters with people in which touchy personal topics are likely to be brought up so that you're not tempted to lie or cause them embarrassment or reveal something you'll later regret. You avoid people with strong prejudices or a fondness for ethnic or racist or sexist jokes so that you don't have to react angrily to their remarks or be ashamed at keeping silent. You avoid associating with others with the same perceived social flaw in order to avoid being identified as one of them. And you avoid being with yourself, left to your own thoughts, so that you don't have to deal with the disturbing issue of why being socially acceptable is more important to you than being who you think you are.

When you can't avoid these uncomfortable situations, you try to manipulate the responses of others to you by draping yourself in a cloak of social respectability.[5] You change your name—Greenberg shortened to "Greene." You change your looks—plastic surgery to deacquilinize a nose, enhance or reduce breasts, remove wattles and wrinkles, or liposuct fat. You use skin lighteners or tanners or cosmetics to hide blemishes and defects. You take speech lessons to overcome unpleasant twangs, malapropisms, and faulty grammar. You adorn yourself with the garb of proper credentials—attendance in the right schools, belonging to the right clubs, knowing the right people. You choose a marriage of convenience as a smokescreen for an unconventional sexual life. You deny your heritage or fabricate your past. Or you may throw yourself into masculine pursuits, such as sexual conquests of women, becoming a war correspondent, or hunting big game, to camouflage your doubts about your manhood.

Wondering whether the image he created of Ernest Hemingway fit all the known facts about him, I asked Scott Donaldson how much he was inventing the person he was trying to bring to life.

"You mean how much truth is there and how much am I making up in my head?" he responded, good-humoredly.

"Well, that's a different way of putting it. I was trying to be polite . . . "

"[The answer is] as little as possible, but I do think that goes on. After all, you're attempting the impossible. We can't know other people or know ourselves, for God's sake. . . . Yet it's an absolutely fascinating process . . . to pretend to do it. There's a certain amount of invention going on, and there has to be. You put six writers/biographers in the same room with the same file cabinet and let them out two weeks later, and you'll get six different responses, and these have to be conditioned by the way that those biographers think and feel. There's no question about it. . . .

"It's kind of amusing that there are all these [books on Hemingway], and that they are so different. Partly it is driven by the market place. So you've got to have a new angle."

"As you've looked at different evidence, has it caused you to change your view of Hemingway?" I pressed. "Has he become a different character in your mind as a result of other information?"

"Maybe a little bit by the publication of the *Garden of Eden*, in which Hemingway reveals what was always there—his androgynous way of looking at love and sex . . . [it probably was always accessible before] . . . men and women who wanted to look exactly alike and change roles. It's very explicit in [that book]."

"So your picture of him has changed with this additional bit of information," I commented, marveling at the irony of how Hemingway, who represented the embodiment of masculinity, should be so preoccupied with how it felt to be a woman or to have sex with a woman who acted and looked like a man. Yet, as Donaldson suggested, Hemingway's concern with castration and tests of masculinity and issues of this sort was always implicit in his writings.

"This is a piece of writing that he never published in his lifetime. It was then edited down drastically. It exists as something like one-fifth of what he left behind. . . . It's a drastically curtailed version of a piece of writing that he did not want published, yet did not destroy. . . . There's a real issue whether such pieces of evidence should be given importance equivalent to books and stories that he did write and did publish."

I agreed with his reservation. But still, Hemingway didn't destroy his manuscript.

Not all people with socially unacceptable propensities subvert what they feel in order to conform to others' expectations. Some find an uneasy accommodation with society by leading secret or double-lives, lives of respectability and duplicity. A successful businessman, for example, wears female clothes whenever he goes out of town. A nun seeks out lesbian relationships outside the convent. An athlete continues to compete even while addicted to cocaine. These are familiar tales. As is usually the case, the secretiveness of this forbidden life, along with the guilt, fear, and excitement it inspires, makes the ordinary lives of these people less dull. It also lets them satisfy different, but irreconcilable aspects of themselves.

John Cheever was a master of deception. As a bisexual, he managed to hide for years his many homosexual affairs from his family and friends, and maintain a public image of utter respectability.

"In your book," I said to Scott Donaldson, "you mentioned Cheever saying that the characters in his fiction began walking into his life rather than his walking into theirs. What did he mean by that?"

"To some extent this happens with all fiction writers. There is a tendency to live in the imagination so much that it overtakes reality. And therefore the people you create in your head become more real than those you meet outside. So it could be simply that kind of process and not necessarily . . . the fragility of the self. . . ."

"The way you portrayed Cheever, the way you saw him, the way you brought him to life, did this differ substantially from how others saw him?"

"Many people saw him differently. In his last years, [he became] a kind of public figure, and so he appears in *People* magazine in a pair of jodhpurs and a riding outfit. He put them on to get his picture taken. He's presenting himself as this kind of country gentleman who rides with hounds. Cheever did not ride horseback. . . . Anybody looking at *People* magazine wouldn't know that. He is constantly falsifying himself."

"Do you see what he did as different from what you or what 'non-writers' do?" I asked

"It's simply more inventive, more interesting, and more compulsive. Cheever could not have behaved otherwise. This was his way of . . . getting along with other people. We all tend to play out parts."

STIGMATIZED LIVES

In the late 1920s, Robert Park, a sociologist, introduced the notion of "marginal" people, whose fate it is to live on the border of two cultures.[6] These people are cultural hybrids, never quite willing to break with their past traditions and never quite accepted into the society in which they seek to find a place. They are part of the cultures in which they live, yet stand apart.

Historically, artists, writers, actors, and musicians have operated on the social fringe, appreciated by a segment of society for their creativity and art, but frowned upon for their lifestyles and deviant values. The notion of social marginality, however, extends beyond professional boundaries. Now it includes any groups of people caught between two cultures, not quite fitting into one and not quite accepted by the other. Many minority or socially disadvantaged groups qualify as being socially marginal. Women who compete in male-dominated professions, Jewish persons who seek acceptance in a predominantly Christian culture, blacks who expect equality in a white society, and homosexuals who proclaim their sexual normality in a mostly heterosexual world—all exist on the social periphery, and all hope to become included within the social center.

While many can carve out a double life or "pass" themselves off as someone they aren't, many socially marginal people don't have this option, especially when physical features or biological and psychological quirks proclaim them as different and somehow undesirable. Because they can't pass, their sense of being different drives them to adopt other kinds of accommodations, which obscure even more who they are.

Take, for instance, "Rafael Johnson," or "Rafe" as he prefers to be called. Rafe is a talented, freelance writer in his forties. He is a natural raconteur and mimic. He's widely read and knowledgeable. He also happens to be an African-American. And being BLACK seems to dominate his consciousness and life. It is his shield and his weapon, and you often aren't sure which is in play. But one thing you know, it represents a barrier between the two of you, even though Rafe makes it seem like it's not—as he regales you and his coterie of whites with harrowing and amusing tales of his ghetto past, told as though he's letting you in on an authentic, black experience. It amuses him to do this, to play on white, liberal guilt, but never enough to make you uncomfortable and defensive since he knows that then you may tire of him. He will say as much when he has had enough to drink.

Yet for all his preoccupation with his blackness, Rafe obviously hungers for acceptance. Only he seems to go about it in a way that makes it unreachable, since he despises the people whom he's able to con into liking him. And since Rafe (the born entertainer who has become a celebrity of sorts among the local elite) knows that he's putting on an act, he never can be sure that it's the "real" Rafe who's being admired, and to make matters worse, by the very people he doesn't like. So what is his self-defeating behavior all about? Even more to the point, where is the real Rafe hiding in this perverse, social game? How do you ever go about finding out?

In his poetry, Langston Hughes repeatedly used the theme of the "tragic mulatto." In his book, *The Souls of Black Folk*, W. E. B. DuBois wrote that blacks possess "no true self-consciousness" but a "double- consciousness," seeing themselves only as perceived by whites through the veil. Because of the struggles of these two people with issues of self and identity, I interviewed Arnold Rampersad, who wrote biographies about both of them.

"You mentioned that Langston Hughes had an unsettled identity. You talked about his repeated use of the theme of the tragic mulatto, about his being caught between two worlds. Did he ever come to peace with himself?" I asked.

"He anchored himself fairly early in certain ways," Professor Rampersad responded. "He anchored himself as a writer. He would not work at any other job but as a writer. Another important anchor was that he would always stay close to the African-American community. He was essentially a very lonely person early in his life, but he identified comfort and love with the regard of the black masses or black community in general. This explains his dedication, also the nature of his poems about the attractiveness of black culture. By the end of his life, he had achieved a certain calm, a certain sense of identity.

"On the other hand, I think that even into the last years of his life there were pools of emptiness within his self, which he knew no one could fill. The loneliness and sense of not belonging were still there, but one of the glories of Hughes as an individual was that he learned early on what to do about what was troubling him. A lot of us never learn. Having learned what to do about it, he did it, and forestalled the chaos and depression.

"What was it he learned to do?" I asked.

"He learned that he could be happy if he wrote for the black American world, and he continued to do that. He kept doing those things because he understood that's what he needed to do, almost as therapy for himself."

"Since you have gathered the most information available on him, I'd like to ask you a hypothetical question. If he were still alive and you were assured that he would answer honestly any of your questions as a biographer, what areas of mystery are still there for you after your two extensive volumes? Is there an unknown part to him that puzzles you?"

"Well I never met him and I never interviewed him. I've gotten most grief from readers about his sexual orientation, and I would have asked him flat out, "Are you gay?" and settled this matter once and for all. But I would also probe him about his attitude to black people. Was this planned? Was this spontaneous? Was the feeling really there? I'd ask him some of the questions that you've been asking me. I'd ask him about the feeling of some people who knew him late in his life that he had developed a kind of callous attitude to other people's pain and suffering . . . a kind of laughing if he heard a misfortune. Where did this come from?"

"When I read your biography, I was looking for mentions of his angst, long periods of depression, wrestling with suicidal thoughts, drinking, and so forth, and I didn't find it. Could you comment on that?" I asked, thinking about the common stereotype of suffering, emotionally unstable poets.

"It's a good question. He had lots of volumes about death. He published a volume, *Dear Lovely Death*. His angst is there, but it did not translate with him into alcoholism, dope, anything like that. Many of his contemporaries in the 1920s did drink too much. It has to be a personal explanation. I believe it has to do with his upbringing. He was a good boy, . . . he was a good man. . . . He was very controlled."

"You made an interesting observation. I think it's an interesting paradox. Here he is a poet, a writer, supposedly going to communicate about his feelings and perceptions, and yet when he undertakes an autobiography, like *The Big Sea*, he hardly reveals anything personal. Do you find that pretty much characterizes his life, that there is both an attempt towards revelation and some kind of barrier?"

"Absolutely, yes. The barrier is there and the self-revelation is there, but only up to a point. I mean, he doesn't reveal that much about himself."

In his now classic work *Stigma*, Erving Goffman describes how a perceived flaw or stigma or handicap—physical, social, or otherwise—often can come to dominate your notion of your self and your interactions with others, becoming the focal point of your identity.[7] You resent this, wanting others to look beyond the socially undesirable quality, yet often don't give them a chance even if they have any inclination to do so. You can't take the risk. So you either show them what you believe they expect to see or only glimpses of you within your social carapace.

You have another dilemma. If you talk about your stigma, you draw more attention to the very feature that mitigates against your social acceptance. And if you don't readily talk about it, you must be ashamed to be who you are: a Jew hiding his Jewishness; an African-American ashamed of his race; an alcoholic denying his problem; or a woman really wanting to be a man. Even if you want to avoid this dilemma entirely, others won't let you.

People naturally dislike being typecast in a role, especially one that places them at a social disadvantage. However, what is psychologically most difficult for them to deal with isn't the real or imagined prejudices of others, which allow their anger toward others to be guilt-free, but their eventually adopting similar prejudices toward themselves and others like them. Because of their social unacceptability, they often begin to view themselves as somehow "defective," much like certain deformed characters in literature. Gregor Samsa, in *The Metamorphosis*, begins to look upon himself as the grotesque creature he has become. Quasimodo the hunchback slinks about, trying to avoid the gaze of others. John Merrick, known as the Elephant Man because of the deformities caused by neurofibromatosis, protests that he is a human being, but he really feels like an animal. When people feel this way, they not only become emotionally imprisoned by their presumed social shortcomings, but after a while they become their own wardens.

No matter how much socially marginal people struggle to arrive at a distinctive understanding of their selves, social forces and their own needs for acceptance conspire to define them in terms of their presumed blemish. Aside from the discrimination and prejudice that this may bring, not all of this stigmatizing process need be psychologically disadvantageous. Once people let themselves become characterized by their race, religion, sexual orientation, gender, or other socially devalued attributes, they are less likely to be confused and tormented about who they are. Their umbrella label offers them a convenient, socially approved way of resolving their ambiguous status and explaining any injustices they perceive.

The tendency of people to identify themselves by means of an all-encompassing social label is reflected in the theme of the One and the Other, which Simone de Beauvoir claims to be the fundamental dilemma for modern feminism.[8] Man is the One and woman is the Other, says de Beauvoir, and this distinction lies at the heart of women's subordinate role to men throughout history. The distinction between the One and the Other applies to many other oppressed or disadvantaged groups as well. And because the members of these groups often have been forced to buy into this invidious distinction—that they are somehow unrepresentative, separate, and different from the more socially privileged rest— they futilely spend their lives in trying to be accepted as a One while believing themselves an Other or in rejecting the status of a One while lauding the virtues of an Other.

A reporter for *People* magazine asked Arthur Ashe whether getting AIDS was the worst burden in his life, and then after he said "No," the reporter asked whether it was his heart attack. "Race has always been my biggest burden," he finally answered. "Having to live as a minority in America."[9]

In his memoir, *Days of Grace,* Ashe talked about how he managed to master the game that all African Americans had to learn of living with reasonable freedom and dignity yet avoiding insult, disappointment, and conflict rooted in racism. "I learned not so much to turn the other cheek as to present, whenever possible, no cheek at all. I learned to give no opportunity for a bigot to pounce on and exploit. I learned in moments of humiliation to walk away with what was left of my dignity, rather than to lose it all in an explosion of rage. I learned to raise my eyes to the high moral ground, and to stake my future on it."[10]

"Do you feel he ever resolved his personal identity before he died and came to some kind of peace?" I asked Professor Arnold Rampersad, who collaborated with Ashe on his autobiography.

"No. He endured his mother's death when he was seven, and it's very hard to know how that got translated into social and political aspects of his character and personality. It clearly made him cool, cold. He talked about seeing his father grieving and openly weeping and so on, and it made him become particularly wary of emotion. But I think he is a person who made his life up in a certain way, drove himself, did what was necessary to be a champion, and then used his reputation to establish himself in certain financial and social ways."

"Do you feel he created his image himself?"

"I know he worked hard at it. He himself would say that. His reputation was everything to him. And I don't think he was ever completely at peace with himself. He was always sorrowful about race in particular, about how he could never be a complete person because of it."

A number of expectations follow when you let yourself become defined by some socially stigmatizing label. Whenever you're with others unlike you, you remain self-conscious and sensitive to what they're thinking about you, expecting that any unintended improprieties on your part will be interpreted as typical of those of your ilk and any of the good qualities as exceptions to the negatively held stereotypes, as in, "For a black, you . . . ," or "For a Jew, you . . . ," or "For a Hispanic, you . . . ," or "For a woman, you . . . ," and so on. Fill in the blank. To avoid these uncomfortable situations, you understandably gravitate toward others with similar persuasions or inclinations, not only for the potential emotional support they can offer but because they often let you redefine your social blemish in more acceptable ways. The very qualities that serve to alienate you from the world around you serve as a bond among those in your group. You no longer need to feel isolated and different. You now have a special status. You belong to a family of fellow sufferers. Alcoholics Anonymous, Take Off Pounds, Recovery, Inc., Depressive and Manic-Depressive Association, Gay Liberation, and countless other groups not only campaign actively for public acceptance but also seek to transform the stigma into a badge of honor by encouraging members to be proud of their heritage and the special outlook their stigma confers. At A.A. meetings, for instance, it's expected that when members get up to speak they first identify themselves as "alcoholic." Many comparable groups encourage their members to openly proclaim what sets them socially apart. During a recent walk in downtown San Francisco, I even encounter a homeless man, collecting money, who wears a large button that reads, "I'm Proud of Being Homeless!"

This tendency for people to proclaim what sets them apart may assume different forms in different settings. As Erving Goffman, the sociologist, so insightfully observes, socially stigmatized people seem to be driven by a "disclosure etiquette."[11] Sometimes they do so in casual but deliberate ways to forestall others from making tactless remarks or displaying their prejudices. Sometimes, to break the ice, they resort to self-deprecatory humor to let others know they aren't unaware of the common stereotypes. Or they may mockingly enact in caricature what they believe others expect of them, showing what otherwise they may easily hide: the shuffling gait, the bowed head and stooped shoulders, the crazy remark, the garishness, the indelicate or rude comment, or any other expected attributes. Or an even more confrontational way of dealing with public attitudes, which lets them take the offensive and maintain the illusion of being in control, is to openly highlight their differences from others and, in doing so, reject others before others can reject them. They make a virtue out of necessity by becoming militant and outspoken. They flout the very stigma, at least symbolically, that sets them apart from the rest: the tattooed butterfly on their shoulder, the earring in one ear lobe, the Star of David, the "butch" haircut, or the right street clothes. Their message to others is, "This is me. Take it or leave it. And if you don't like it, then screw you. I couldn't care less."

Instances of this are endless.

I offer a guest a cocktail at my home and he declines, saying he can't drink, he's an alcoholic, and, as the rest of us drink, he makes his past drinking excesses and his present abstinence the unwanted topic of our conversation.

At a recent social gathering, I try to engage a young instructor in conversation about his research but instead find myself listening to his account of his own experiences as a black.

On a TV variety show, a relatively unknown comedian with an exaggerated Yiddish accent spices his spiel with painfully tasteless ethnic jokes about his family.

A young friend shaves off her long hair as an act of feminine liberation in order to avoid all sexual attention by men but now draws even more attention from everyone.

I attend a computer seminar and the instructor laces his lecture with comments about his shortness, which is not what I notice beforehand and isn't what I come there to hear about.

There are legions of people who understandably feel compelled to make declarations of this sort, people who at various points in their lives choose to liberate themselves from their invisible or obvious social restraints and live within the self-imposed constraints of their newly visible roles. These displays often have a paradoxical impact on me, which, I suspect, is different from what these people intend. In all these instances, I'm mostly interested in these individuals' knowledge and work and not their difficulties with their skin color, their religion, their height, their sexuality, or their drinking problems. But if I'm oblivious to or dimly aware of these characteristics before, they dominate my consciousness thereafter. No doubt they are all eager for approval and acceptance, but their entire manner emphasizes their differentness and drops an invisible wall between us. I want to establish contact with them, but I find I'm put off by their covert, paradoxical message: "I want to be recognized for me, for my intelligence, my personality, my talents, and not be discriminated against because I'm socially undesirable, so to make my point I won't let you forget I'm socially undesirable!" Instead of defining themselves by the myriad of attributes they share in common with others or perhaps by the most meaningful distinction among human beings, their "character"—namely, whether they are decent, friendly, perceptive, empathetic, generous, truthful, or reliable—they focus on the differences that aren't prized in their prevailing culture and unintentionally accentuate their sense of social alienation.

THUMBING ONE'S NOSE

Let's take this seeming paradox one step further. It's easy to understand why people exposed to discrimination should feel alienated from society. It's also understandable why many, almost as an overcompensation, should rebel against this prejudice and proudly trumpet their differentness. But it's hard to understand why many who potentially can avoid being discriminated against should exaggerate their social differentness and thereby seem to invite others to stigmatize them.

Over a period of a month, I happen to read three biographies of gay men.[12] By the time I put the last book down, I'm struck by a remarkable coincidence. All of these men, even as youths, accentuated rather than hid feminine characteristics even though they experienced grief and ridicule for it.

Truman Capote, with his high-pitched voice, daintiness, and effeminacy, endured the ridicule of other children even though later, with his remarkable ability for story-telling, he came to be regarded as their mascot. Oscar Wilde, perhaps protected more from this early ridicule by his favored upbringing and station in life, still flaunted his differentness by his feminine gestures, and even, later in life, seemed to provoke being convicted and jailed for his proclivities. As a child, Henry Faulkner, a little known Kentucky artist with a primitive, Rousseau-type style, applied lipstick and rouge to his face, subjecting himself to the ridicule of his schoolmates and the embarrassment of his foster mother, who dragged him from doctor to doctor to rectify the problem. Sickly, nervous and high-strung, he spent hours in the woods alone drawing pictures, even though his mother thought they were the Devil's work. As he got older, he wore makeup openly, sometimes dressed in drag, and strutted like a rooster down the street, often accompanied by Alice, his bourbon-drinking goat.

As I puzzle over this matter, I realize that the early, exaggerated effeminacy in these persons is not uncommon. Andy Warhol wore makeup and had effeminate characteristics. Cecil Beaton, the photographer, put on lipstick as a child and showed an inordinate interest in fashion. Mark Blitzstein, the composer, displayed feminine gestures. These instances go on and on. These individuals are clearly different from other children, but compared to each other, are remarkably the same.

What is so intriguing about their behavior is that it apparently contradicts the rules of learning theory, which hold that people tend to act in ways that get praise or reward and avoid censure or punishment. This certainly isn't so for the three individuals in question, who, if anything, brazenly flaunted their different-ness even at the cost of being heckled by others. Put differently, they seemed to invite the ridicule they got.

How to make sense of this parody of femininity: the limp wrists, the shifting hips, the sashaying walk, and the cultivated mannerisms? How to make sense of the stubborn resistance of these individuals, even as children, to the sometimes extreme measures taken by their parents or teachers or others to make "real" boys or men of them—not only their resistance to these pressures but often their per-verse exaggeration of the offending gestures? How to make sense of their need to shock others and be the center of attention even from an early age? Can this pos-sibly be biologically determined, something these individuals can do nothing about, a predisposition they are obliged to express? But I find it hard to imagine a gene that produces feminine characteristics in caricature—characteristics far in excess of what their potential role models, their mothers and sisters, display or their cultures dictate.

The convenient way to explain this away is to say that they behave that way for attention—perhaps a way to counter their sensed, personal "invisibility." Their peculiarities and dramatic flair insure that everybody will notice. Sure, but why flaunt their flaws, the characteristics that make them appear different? If they hunger for attention, why don't they do those things that parents, teachers and other children expect of them so that they can become popular and admired? I suppose that in some obscure way these persons could be trying to express their perceived differentness from others, which they sense is in the direction of femininity, and under the urge to do this, overshoot the mark. Or are their actions smokescreens for something else, a bid for personal validation, perhaps, or an infantile desire for total acceptance from adoring parental figures (or "society"), who will continue to love them unconditionally despite their mis-behavior?

Yet another possible reason for these burlesque portrayals of femininity is that they represent a kind of self-mocking humor, which disarms potential adver-saries by taking the offensive. By lampooning themselves, they keep others from harpooning them. Capote was self-mocking in his antics, possibly full of self-hatred, because he absorbed the stigma so completely. Oscar Wilde made a par-ody of his dandyism. And Henry Faulkner, with his goat and other bizarre behavior, made a mockery out of convention. As seductive as this explanation is, it still falls short. It doesn't account for the existence of these behaviors from their early youth, when a self-deprecatory humor was unlikely to exist. And it doesn't explain why they should advertise their social stigma in bold relief when they presumably are able to conceal it.

The glimmer of an answer comes to me one day as I jog shirtless in an isolated field, dressed in my Speedo swimsuit. I have just finished reading a biography about Janis Joplin and wonder what perversity caused her to be so taunting, so provocative and flamboyant in almost every aspect of her life. My thoughts switch to a farm auction nearby that will be held in a couple of hours. There are a few items there that I plan to bid on. I visualize myself nonchalantly standing there in the crowd incongruously wearing only my brief bathing suit and my Australian bush hat, and acting perfectly normal. I savor the image of these mostly proper, God-fearing country folk trying to act as though nothing is amiss as we exchange pleasantries between auction bids while obviously shocked by my sartorial breach of decorum. It tickles me to imagine what they will say about me afterwards, "That crazy university professor!" I relish the notion that I will be the topic of conversation within the county for days to come.

I set these exhibitionistic thoughts aside, but not before I get an inkling about what impels Janis Joplin to act as she does. It's not just the attention she wants, I realize, judging by my own reaction, since despite my fleeting fantasy I can't care less whether the onlookers at the auction, most of whom I don't know, are aware of me or not. What prompts this perverse fantasy in me—and perhaps it is the very same nemesis as in all people who feel different—is entirely different. Because I never can blend in and be accepted completely by these country folk, I want to shock them with my differentness to let them know I don't care. It's symbolically like thumbing my nose at them.

What potential social or biological value can this seemingly provocative behavior serve? I search for other instances of such perverse behavior in Nature or society. The image of a squirrel taunting a dog comes to mind. Then I remember Pavlov's studies and his observation that certain dogs resist being conditioned, sometimes even showing opposite responses. Among humans, certain Indian groups create special roles for "contraries," people who seem constitutionally disposed to defy tribal customs. Within most societies, mavericks, renegades, dissidents, and rebels challenge tradition and push the limits, often at great personal risk. Could there be parallels between the need to exaggerate per-ceived differentness and contrary behavior of this sort? If so, then the ultimate paradox exists. The very differentness that most societies try to squelch in order to preserve stability may be their necessary life blood, capable of preventing the potential stagnation and decay that homogeneity and conformity can bring. Peo-ple who blatantly and persistently thwart conventions may be a ferment for social progress. As "social mutants," so to speak, they may force their prevailing culture to accommodate greater diversity and broaden its boundaries for social acceptability, thereby conceivably enriching the culture, if they aren't suppressed or eliminated first.

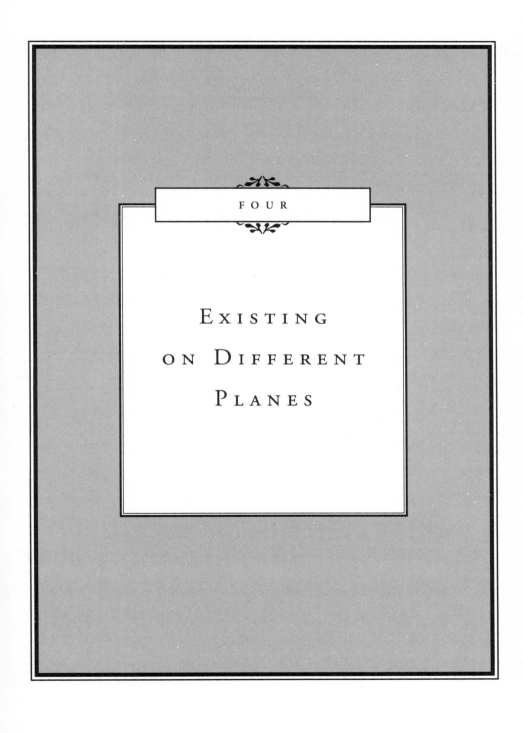

FOUR

EXISTING
ON DIFFERENT
PLANES

CAN OTHERS KNOW US BETTER than we know ourselves?
During a morning walk, I silently rate how well I know myself, then ask my wife to rate how well she knows me on a scale from zero to one hundred percent. I estimate I know myself seventy five percent; she says she knows me ninety percent. "That's ridiculous, you can't know me better than I know myself," I protest, thinking about my private and often taboo thoughts. "But I do," she replies. Annoyed, I blurt out, "Now why did I ask such a stupid question?" She smiles, then says, "Do you want me to tell you?"

This anecdote highlights a number of important issues. By initially asking my wife to rate her knowledge of me, I make the assumption that the real me, my essence, is represented by the sanctum sanctorum of my private mental life, which, unless I choose to reveal it, is inaccessible to all. By her response, she makes the assumption that knowledge about my secret and forbidden thoughts is irrelevant to her knowledge of me. Whatever the reasons, I find it disturbing that someone can claim to know me even better than I know myself. It's a threat to my sense of autonomy. The only consolation I have is that I'm in good company. After his wife made a similar claim, John Cheever lamented in his journal, "It seems so unnatural."[1]

In general, what we mean by knowing ourselves is an awareness of our own mental processes that may or may not precede any action, or in the absence of this awareness, knowledge of the mental processes that may or may not follow any action, letting us reconstruct for ourselves why the action happened. It is our awareness of these mental processes (whether or not they actually are necessary for these actions) that sustains our belief in personal options and freedom of choice. We reason that if our thoughts and behaviors are linked, then they must be causally related, especially if one precedes the other. We resist the possibility that our thought processes may simply represent *ad hoc* justifications or *post hoc* rationalizations for doing what we're inclined to do, accentuating our performances like accompanists at a recital.

Since those who believe they know us can't read our thoughts unless we reveal them, they have to rely on other clues about us. We may experience our actions as purposeful, but others often perceive them as dispositional traits that determine how predictable we are. The implications of this are important. If we are completely predictable to others, then we represent nothing more than biological servomechanisms, automatically responding to environmental stimuli according to our instincts or psychological programming. Total predictability means strict causality, and strict causality means the lack of free will. When there are no surprises, then strict cause-and-effect or stimulus-response must be at work, negating the theoretical existence of a sovereign, independent, and potentially spontaneous self.

I tell my wife that she is probably bored being married to someone so predictable. She wisely denies that, saying it's comforting to her to know how I will behave. Then she offers a sop to my ego by saying that anyway I'm not totally predictable. On rare occasions I can surprise her.

BEHAVIORAL FORECASTING

Fortunately for my pride, the issue of being totally predictable is more theoretical than real, probably because all the relevant variables about people never can be known. No matter how well we know others, they always have the potential for some unexpected, out-of-character response, if not in action then in their fantasies or thoughts. For example, a farmer who engages in the same routine day in and day out, attends church regularly and does whatever he is supposed to do, one day goes in the barn and, in Richard Cory fashion, puts a bullet through his head. A former member of the Ku Klux Klan and a strict Baptist like William O. Black, after appointment to the Supreme Court, turns out to be one of its most liberal members. Lovers who at one time are willing to die for one another later turn out to be bitter enemies. Once sentenced to prison, a White House aide becomes a born-again Christian.

Predictability, then, is less of an absolute than a probability statement, much like weather forecasting. Knowing others, in one sense, means that we're able to make reasonable guesses about how they are disposed to act: their habits, their customary responses, and their typical patterns of behavior under varying circumstances. When they are capricious, volatile, or unstable, they keep us emotionally off-balance. The more important others are to us, the more important it is for us to know what to expect from them. So when they don't behave as we expect them to, we try to find ways to increase the accuracy of our forecasts.[2] One of the ways we do this is to construct plausible narratives to explain their behavior.

THE "WHY" BEHIND THE "WHAT"

If we presume to know others, what they think, say, and do must make sense.[3] There must be a rationale for their behavior, no matter how impulsive or erratic it seems. The key to understanding them, then, is to discern what their motivations are, or at least what seen or unseen forces prompt their actions.

When I questioned Joan Peyser about how she could be sure that her biographical portraits of people like Leonard Bernstein or George Gershwin were true, she told me, "Before I sit down to write, I spend at least a year learning enough about my subject to allow me to put into one sentence what I believe his inner agenda is. By that I mean: what does he have to do in his life in addition to his external, artistic goals. This is something the person rarely articulates to himself. It is something on an unconscious level that often has to do with a parent or sibling. If he is an artist, it is that which will drive him relentlessly. Once I put that goal down on paper, everything in the life and work falls into place. What I have learned is that each of us is at the least consistent. There are never any surprises. If the biographer understands the life in this way, he or she never thinks: 'I would never have believed my subject could do this.'"

It's reasonable to assume that once we identify the real motives of people, we have come to understand them. The problem is how to be sure that these motives are their real ones. Do we ask these people? But what if they don't know what drives them? Do we ask others who know them? But the perceptions of others may be biased. Or do we simply guess at what their motives are? If so, how do we know we're right? In a fascinating discussion of why Van Gogh cut off his ear, William Runyan offers guidance on this matter.[4] Although his comments have to do with judging the reliability of different biographical accounts, they apply equally well to how we know others.

During the course of his research, Runyan identified thirteen separate accounts about why Vincent Van Gogh cut off the lower half of his left ear in 1888 and entrusted it to a prostitute, asking her to "keep this object carefully." One source said that Van Gogh's act of self-mutilation represented a symbolic self-castration, stemming from thwarted homosexual impulses toward Gauguin. Another source said that he was influenced by the bullfights he saw in Arles in which the victorious matador received the ear of the bull as a reward. Yet another argued that this was an act of penance, designed to win his mother's love. Still another source said that this was a way to get his brother, Theo, to care for him rather than spend Christmas with his fiancée. Another source said that he was trying to recreate the Bible scene in the Garden of Gethsemane in which Simon Peter cut off the ear of Malchus, a servant of a high priest, who had come to seize Christ. Another source said Van Gogh cut off his ear in an attempt to silence the disturbing auditory hallucinations he was experiencing during a psychotic episode. The explanations go on, each source convinced of the correctness of its view.

For our purposes, the matter of which of these explanations is the correct one is irrelevant. The issue has to do with how to go about identifying the most plausible one. Runyan lists six criteria. The explanation should be logically sound. It should be comprehensive enough to explain any puzzling aspects of the event in question. It should have sufficient predictive value and survive the challenge of any contradictions. It should accommodate the full range of available evidence. It should be consistent with more general knowledge about human behavior. And it should be more credible than the competing hypotheses.

Though Runyan's criteria bring a semblance of scientific rigor to an otherwise murky area, they offer false reassurance. Since the ultimate test of any explanation becomes its credibility, then no absolute judgement about its validity ever can be made. The reason is that what is credible to some people may not be to others, no matter the nature or extent of the evidence. At least, that is one lesson we can draw from the many convincing accounts of Marilyn Monroe.

As for Van Gogh's mutilated ear, it isn't simply our inability to question him directly that keeps us from understanding his bizarre act. Even if we had been able to ask him why he lopped off his ear, his account, however believable, wouldn't settle the matter. If he told us that he did it because God commanded him to, for example, or because of his disturbing hallucinatory voices or for some other reason, we still couldn't tell whether he was right, whether he believed he was right, or whether he was lying. The reason is we have no objective way to establish the "truth" of his account. Plausibility becomes our only basis for judgment. Though it creates the illusion of understanding and causality, it isn't synonymous with truth. Therefore, what someone regards as the most plausible explanation for certain events may actually be the least probable.

The case of Linda Gray Sexton, the daughter of Anne Sexton, the poet, illustrates this well. In her autobiography, Linda Sexton described many of the traumas she endured while growing up.[5] When she was an infant, her mother, by her own confession, tried to choke her several times to stop her crying. As a child, ashamed and trying not to see, she watched her mother many times, naked from the waist down, masturbating in her presence. What was perhaps the hardest experience for her to forgive (as Diane Middlebrook, the biographer of Anne Sexton, told me was also hardest for her to forgive in her subject) was her mother forcing her to have sex when she was about twelve years old. Even after years of psychotherapy, Linda Sexton kept reexperiencing this terrible memory whenever her husband wanted sex. "I sometimes come back to that dark night when my mother's sticky body lay tightly on mine," she writes, "the stink of her booze breath, the legacy of fear and self-hatred with which she left me." But forgive her she does, probably because her mother meant so much to her in so many other ways. As often happens with child sexual abuse victims, the way she was able to excuse her mother years after her suicide was by first blaming herself, realizing that when her mother climbed on top of her, she didn't push her off and scream (largely because she wanted to please her mother). As for why her mother subjected her to this horrible ordeal at all, the daughter, now claiming emotional reconciliation with the memory of her mother, believes that her mother couldn't help herself because *she was mentally ill*. She finds solace in this seemingly plausible explanation, even though it explains nothing at all. Countless people with mental illness don't emotionally and sexually abuse their children.

Even biographers sometimes need to make the behavior of their subjects more plausible so that they can continue to feel positively toward them. During my interview with Roxana Robinson, she mentioned that she came across a couple of things about Georgia O'Keeffe that she initially found hard to forgive. I asked her to elaborate.

"There was a moment when O'Keeffe was in her late twenties, and she was introduced to a niece of Alfred Stieglitz, who was then three or four years old, and the niece had been told what to do when she met this woman, and she stepped forward and curtsied and said, 'I'm glad to meet you, Aunt Georgia.' Her memory of it was that Georgia stepped forward and slapped her in the face and said, 'Never call me Aunt Georgia.' I find that a shocking act. But at the time O'Keeffe was under terrible pressure from Stieglitz's family. She was very unhappy at his summer house, surrounded by his relatives and surrounded by behavior that she did not approve of. And she also was very anxious about the issue of being married, and felt very unhappy that she had given up her own single, independent status. In fact, I now can't remember if she was married when she did this. It was important for me to unravel the roots of that (irrational and cruel) act. But when you reveal her as a woman on the edge of a nervous breakdown, someone who was unsure of herself, very anxious about her power and her identity at that time, it becomes less shocking."

"Did you know about this before you undertook the biography?" I asked, wondering why it was so necessary for Robinson to excuse her subject.

"Yes. One of the reasons that I [undertook the biography was to correct the public image of her that mostly had to do with the last twenty years of her life]. She was an old woman. She was past her years of great work. She was very resentful of public intrusions into her life. She was tart-tongued and difficult, and every time there would be an article that mentioned her, you would see a picture of this ancient crone-like woman and a quote which was unpleasant. And looking at the work, which is passionate and warm and emotionally accessible, it seemed terrible to me that this was the image that was being left in the minds of the public after this woman's life. I wanted to reveal the woman who had produced the work, which was radiant and ingenuous and powerful and full of passion."

I sympathized with Robinson's intent.[6] After all, this wasn't so dissimilar from what Linda Sexton tried to do with her mother or, for that matter, what most of us do when we search for mitigating reasons that let us remain positively disposed toward those who abuse us. Plausibility becomes the servant of our needs, not the master of our will.

THREE LEVELS OF BEING

So far we've found that knowing others depends on being able to predict with reasonable accuracy their responses under different circumstances and being able to explain them in a convincing way. But knowing others in this way says nothing about knowing them in their different modes of existence. As it happens, people simultaneously exist on three separate planes for us—as persons generically, as people with personal identities, and as distinct individuals—and who they are for us at any moment depends on what we want to know about them and what vantage point we take.

GENERIC BEINGS

At the most fundamental level, people exist generically as human beings, and as such, share many features in common. They have similar biological drives and basic psychological needs and respond to the same sorts of social pressures. They may be absolute strangers, specks on a distant landscape, faces in the crowd, but we may know them well enough in an abstract sense to predict certain of their behaviors with a reasonable degree of accuracy and explain why they act as they do.

Various social organizations exploit this generic information about people for different purposes. As abstract entities—taxpayers, home owners, heads of households, deployable troops, viewing audiences, drivers, or accident victims—people can be identified by their social security numbers, credit card numbers, serial numbers, personal identification numbers, driver licenses, or dog tags. They represent figures, points on a curve, survey statistics, or census data, which can be transformed into base rates, frequencies, distributions, or bar graphs that reveal important characteristics about them and predict certain patterns and trends. Their entire value or meaning as humans derives from whatever purpose they serve for those collecting this information on them. As examples, political scientists, epidemiologists, psychologists, researchers, advertisers, military leaders, tax collectors, and others who deal with humans in this generic fashion, use this information to predict their voting tendencies, buying patterns, casualty rates, health care practices, product preferences, or other behaviors, and construct theories to explain them. Beyond that all other personal information about what these people think, feel, or do during the course of their lives is superfluous.

Existing on this conceptual plane, people remain human but dehumanized. This distinction lets leaders of various political, scientific, military, or social agencies make strategic decisions that affect the populace at large without having to deal with the preferences of particular groups or the desires of individual people. Decisions about risk-benefit ratios, cost effectiveness, acceptable casualty rates or body counts, expected dropout frequencies, acceptable noncompliance rates, and appropriate unemployment rates are all derivative from this mentality.

While we may have no professional interest in this way of knowing people, we have a strong personal stake in it. In fact, this is how we relate to most of humanity, but in a less focused way. We acknowledge our biological, psychological, and emotional commonality with all other people, but beyond that they exist as abstractions for us, as we do for them. Knowing others mostly in this remote way offers important psychological advantages, not only because our brains lack the capacity to process specific information about several billion other people but because we would be emotionally and cognitively incapacitated if it could. As long as others are part of the unknown masses, they exist for us in the realm of ideas. This shields us from overidentifying with them when we learn about the tragedies that befall them, such as earthquakes, famines, or wars, or the adverse political or economic forces they are subjected to. At this plane of their existence, they remain real for us but have no individual reality.

BRAND NAMES

It's not sufficient for us to see others as generic persons similar to all other human beings and let it go at that. We possess an urge for classification that makes us want to seek commonalities with certain people and differences with others. As a result, we categorize ourselves and others according to such characteristics as social class, race, gender, education, marriage, parenthood, religion, political ideology, profession, physical stature, special failings, or affiliations with various groups.[7] These characteristics contribute to our sense of knowing others and our own sense of personal identity. And in many instances, they become shorthand representations of them and us.

Since the labels we attach to people contain implicit information about their likely attitudes and values, they offer us a way of predicting and interpreting their actions. As condensed packets of information, these labels are mentally economical and relatively resistant to change.[8] Much like uniforms that teams and armies wear, they let us know instantly if others are friends or foes, where they stand on various issues, what their roles are, and whether they are trustworthy or not. They become essential social apparel. As soon as others strip them off, we paste them back on.[9] Labeling is so ingrained in the way we see people that even biographers, attempting to bring their subjects to life, rely heavily on labels to establish their identities and even sometimes to explain the nature of their artistic works.

Joan Peyser, the biographer of such musical greats as George Gershwin and Leonard Bernstein, offered important insights on how the religious, ethnic, and national identities of her subjects shaped their sense of self and their creative expression as well.

"The more the artist knows who he is, the greater the artist he can be," she informed me. "Gershwin knew he was an American. He also knew he was a Jew. And he created songs that compare to those by Schubert. Bernstein, on the other hand, was conflicted as an American and as a Jew. While he appeared, at the start of his career, to be the prototypical American, he signed, in the '30s, '40s and '50s, countless Communist documents. And, in the '60s, he supported the Black Panthers, a militant organization bent on killing American policemen and dynamiting public facilities. Similarly Bernstein's Jewishness was at cross purposes with itself. In the '40s, after the War of Independence in Israel, he became the conductor of the Israel Philharmonic, directing concerts in Jerusalem, Tel Aviv, Haifa and Beersheba. Yet in 1945, when Moyshe

Koussevitzky, the great cantor who had been in concentration camps in Poland, sang at a synagogue on Yom Kippur, Bernstein bolted out at the end, announcing he was off to a great Italian dinner, flouting the notion of fasting. These mixed signals never ceased. In the '70s and '80s, Bernstein made known his activities in the Arab section of Israel as well as his pro-Arab political stance whenever he went to that country to conduct.

"It was partly because of this absence of identity that Bernstein was able to blend into the head of any composer whose work he conducted and that, in combination with his musicianship, made him a truly remarkable conductor. But he never wrote great music on his own. He never became a creative artist of the magnitude of Gershwin."

While labels give useful information about others, especially about the nature of their biological, psychological, and social identities, they also serve as a basis for stereotyping and typecasting. Once we pigeonhole others, we seldom can be proven wrong. When their actions conform to our expectations, they confirm them. When they don't, they represent exceptions to the rule. Because of this, labels may create a false sense of knowing others better than we do. They offer self-fulfilling prophesies that support what we're already inclined to believe.

Not all labeling, though, need be biased. There are ways of safeguarding against this. For instance, by comparing the characteristics of one group of people with another, we can scientifically test whether true differences exist between them. Various statistical analyses are available to establish if any observed differences are "significant" or merely due to chance. We also have recourse to mathematical models that let us evaluate the extent to which certain responses can be predicted. But the one restriction of these analyses and whatever conclusions we reach based on them is that they apply only to groups as a whole, not to any of its individual members. On this plane of their existence, individuals hold little reality for us other than as members of certain groups.

SINGULAR INDIVIDUALS

While certain labels may convey useful information about people, especially about the nature of their biological, professional, and social identities, they often are misleading because of what they don't say. This is especially so if we maintain that each person is unique. Beyond their personal identities, people display all sorts of idiosyncratic or singular behaviors. They also are more or less outgoing, funny, questioning, innovative, eccentric, talented, or something-or-other than others. They may conform to certain stereotypes, but they also show particular traits that set them apart. For Brendan Gill, the biographer of such celebrities as Frank Lloyd Wright, Tullulah Bankhead, and Charles Lindbergh, these traits constitute their basic nature, their authentic self. "Everybody has a self, a quiddity," Gill told me, "but you can have a self without having an identity." With this outlook, the essence of a person is not defined by a collage of identifying labels, which contribute to his or her personal identity, but by his or her innate and often distinctive traits.

Whether these distinctive traits define the true essence of a person is a matter of debate. But what there can be little argument about is that each individual has distinctive traits. These distinctive traits represent a person's personal signature, fingerprints, or particular markings. Knowing people in this way means being aware of their twitches, mannerisms, ways of speaking, cognitive styles, quirks, idiosyncrasies, and the emotional motifs and leitmotifs that govern their lives. These features bring them into sharper focus. In their extreme, they sometimes serve as a basis for caricature. When incorporated in anecdotes, they offer mental snapshots of the person, which we store in the photo albums of our mind. Like contrived poses for photographs, when the photographer tells us to smile or say "cheese," each of these images conveys something special about the person, containing its own implicit moral or story.

I asked Victor Bockris about his techniques for instilling life in his subjects, such as William Burroughs, Andy Warhol, and Keith Richards.

"The way I do it is to let them talk quite a lot in my books. I try and have a lot of quotes from the actual person, the subject of the book, because the way they speak is a voice portrait. The syntax and the words they choose and the things they harp on tell you a lot about them in quite an intimate manner. I am like a photographer. My book is in a sense hundreds and hundreds of photographs cut up like David Hockney, montages of images that are just done in writing. For example, if I interview somebody in Philadelphia who knew Andy Warhol in 1955, and I take away a tape recording of two hours, which is about eighty typed pages, in that eighty pages are going to be a number of word photographs. The person is going to say something like, "I was in a restaurant with Andy one time when he brought out some chocolate kisses and put them on the table and gave them to the waiter, and then he got up and gave the waiter a $5 bill and walked out." That's a photograph. So that will probably go into the book verbatim. So I'm snipping out photographs from interviews, putting them into the book, and then, of course, weaving them into the text."

However well we believe we know particular people, we never can know them well unless we can tell how they will act under different conditions and why they act as they do. If we don't know them in different contexts, we may have trouble telling whether their actions are due to chance, are characteristic for a specific situation, or are invariant responses to a wide variety of conditions.

This raises again the niggling matter of my wife's claim of knowing me better than I know myself, which triggered this entire discussion. Obviously, in making this claim, she was not referring to knowing me as a generic being or as a composite of labels, since certain experts with access to my demographic characteristics, physical attributes, and group affiliations may be able to predict and explain many of my responses on these planes of my existence far better than she. She meant knowing me in a singular way—my peculiarities and bents. But my dilemma is how to reconcile her claim with my proprietary rights to my own experiences and my awareness of what motivates me. If her knowledge of me is greater than mine, then I may be deceiving myself about how well I know myself.

What we need is an impartial way to settle this matter. Already, we have seen that on other planes of people's existence there exist objective ways to know them better. As generic beings, they represent simple statistics, numbers, or data, whose responses can be counted and tabulated to document trends and establish base rates, which then can be used to make predictions and generate explanations. As brand names or collections of labels, people also exist as members of particular groups, whose frequency, amount, and range of responses can be statistically compared to those of other groups to learn if significant differences exist. But what can we do on the singular plane of people's existence to objectively test how well we know them?

Though not foolproof, a practical way to do this suggests itself. The best way for me to tell whether there is any merit in my wife's claim about knowing me better than I know myself is to figure out which of us has been in a more advantageous position to gather objective information about the way I'm disposed to act in different situations. An A-B-A-B model, often used in single case studies to test how a subject responds to particular conditions, suits this purpose well.[10] With the A-B-A-B model, the observer (in this case, my wife or I) first ascertains how I act under standard conditions (A), then how I act when new variables are introduced (B), then how I act when the standard conditions are restored (A), and lastly how I act after reintroduction of the new variables (B). If the observer notes that I consistently show certain patterns of behavior during condition B that differ from those I show during condition A, then he or she presumably knows something characteristic about me. Naturally, with this model of knowing, knowing me in any depth involves knowing how I'll respond under many different A-B-A-B conditions.

As it happens, in real life we aren't in a position to systematically expose people we hope to know to a series of A-B-A-B conditions, so we never can learn about all their typical response patterns. However, over the course of time, we sometimes have a chance to accumulate information about them during many unplanned, natural "experiments" that simulate these conditions. With some perceptiveness on our part, we may come to identify certain of their tendencies.

As for which of us—my wife or I—is better situated to identify my tendencies with this particular model, my wife seems to have a decided advantage over me. She has been able to observe me informally over the years under countless A-B-A-B-type conditions and learn how I'm disposed to act under each. When I try to observe myself, I only can do so retrospectively as an imaginary observer by watching mental playbacks of my experiences. I don't have my wife's capacity for direct, detached, on-the-spot examinations of me since I am too busy being who I am and have a vested interest in remaining so. In these impromptu, natural experiments, I'm stuck in the role of the subject, mostly interpreting my decisions and actions as initiated by me rather than prompted by external forces. Because of this, I keep experiencing myself anew, despite the number of times I may have been in a particular situation before. She has the vantage point of the experimenter, empirically collecting data on me and comparing responses in different situations. By contextualizing my actions, she is better able to detect any outside influences on me. Therefore, if the A-B-A-B model represents our most objective way to know someone on his or her singular plane of existence, I'm forced to conclude that my wife probably knows me better than I know myself. So what does that tell me? It says that if I'm truly interested in learning more about me, I need to learn how others see me. But to do so, I need to shift my perspective of me from a strictly autobiographical to a more biographical one.

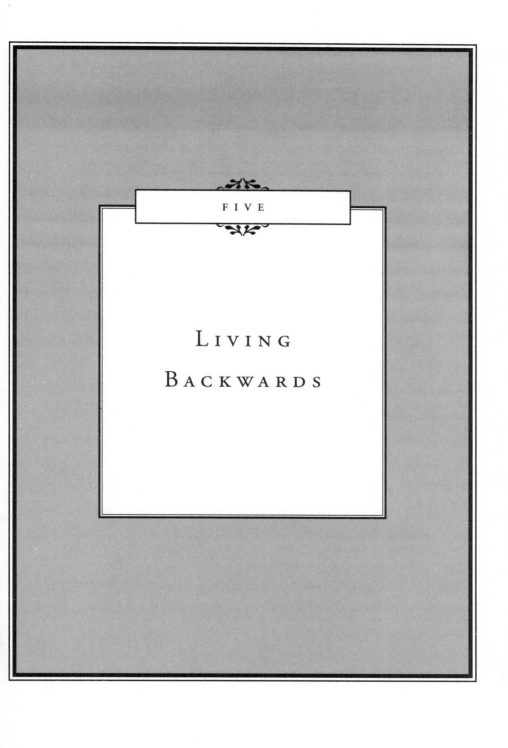

FIVE

LIVING
BACKWARDS

According to the biographer Christopher Benfey, Stephen Crane lived out events in his imagination long before he experienced them in reality.[1] Contrary to expectations that a writer's works are based on past experiences, he actually wrote about events before he experienced them, making his fiction eerily predictive of what lay ahead. For instance, his only experiences with battle, as a highly paid war correspondent, came years after he published his novel about the Civil War, *The Red Badge of Courage*, acclaimed worldwide for its vivid portrayal of war. He wrote *Maggie*, his novel about a prostitute, long before he fell in love with a real-life madam. Some time after writing several stories about shipwrecks, he actually found himself aboard a foundering steamer. In his novel, *The Third Violet*, he wrote about courting a society belle; later, he carried out a courtship with one through his letters. To dismiss these instances as coincidental cases of life imitating art is to overlook the full implications of Crane's experiences. In a metaphorical sense, he seemed to be living his life backwards, experiencing the future before it happened.

I asked Christopher Benfey, "In what way was Stephen Crane's double life different from that of others?"

"In Crane's case, the relation between the life imagined and the life lived struck me as so literal and extreme and almost lock-step that he seemed a particularly good example of *lived doubleness* that I think is common to just about everyone."

"Why do you think he did that? Why did he have to translate his fantasies into reality?"

"If I were required to sketch out what such a motivation would be, I could give two parts of it pretty quickly, and the third part might still need a good deal of psychological expertise. The first two are cultural. Crane grew up in a household that was intensely religious and intensely involved with a fairly literal interpretation of the Bible. His father was a Methodist minister. All of his uncles on his mother's side were Methodist ministers. His grandfather was, and so on. One tenet of a certain kind of nineteenth-century evangelical Christianity is that you model your life on the Good Book. So the idea of living his life according to an earlier script could not be more deeply ingrained in Crane's temperament.

"The second thing is that Crane lived in a journalistic culture, in addition to the religious culture . . . that tended to frame the story first and then go out and try to find it. Crane's letters are full of requests to cover the next streetcar strike or to write a certain kind of story before the event actually happened. He also worked for people like Hearst whose basic view was that if you didn't have the news story that you needed, you went out and tried to create it. There is some evidence that Hearst did engineer the sinking of the battleship *Maine* in order to get the U.S. involved in the Spanish American War.

"So those are two parts of what I would think of as a three part motivation. . . . The third is tougher. [It has to do with] the reason for the particular extremity and literalness of Crane's write-it-then-live-it temperament, and I don't really see a way to go much further with that, except by finding other temperaments who seem the same way and trying to see what they might have in common. This is a character type that you sometimes run into with writers."

Does this mean that you actually live portions of your life backwards with future experiences preceding present ones, like the rewinding of a videotape? Of course not. Your inexorable progression through successive developmental stages insures that you will move forward in time until your biological clock winds down. What it means more exactly is that you exhibit what Christopher Benfey called "lived doubleness," meaning that you simultaneously live in your imagination and in the real world, even though these experiences may not be in synch. When the imagined experiences you explicitly think about, write about, or express in other ways come true, they create the illusion of a reversal in time. Because the future comes to be experienced before it actually happens, it takes on aspects of the past.

The notion that you, like Crane, may experience portions of your life in a reverse order raises important questions about the nature of the self. From an experiential standpoint, what if all you take for granted about the temporal course of your life is the other way around, and your life represents not so much a progression into the future as a realization of the past? This has a ring of science fiction about it. Instead of building your life only on past experiences, you actually may be living your life to conform to stories already written for you. If you aren't a novelist, like Crane, your stories may be vague and inchoate, without clear narrative structure, but stories nonetheless, waiting for you to live them. Much of what you do in life—maturing, selecting a mate, procreating, exhibiting certain temperaments, aging—may be written in your genes in a language you don't yet know how to decode, creating erosions and gullies over the unexplored terrain of your life through which your life story flows. Perhaps much of what you strive to become is already preordained for you by your biological predisposition, inculcated in you by your parents, suggested by cultural myths, or spelled out in places like the New Testament. Perhaps you spend your life seeking experiences that you're supposed to have and that feel "right" because they are indelibly written on your mind in an invisible script. If this be so, then over the course of your life, you simply become what you're destined to be.

Lest this discussion seem too hypothetical, let's turn to certain examples from real life. William Manchester, the biographer of such notables as John F. Kennedy, Winston Churchill, Douglas MacArthur, H. L. Mencken, and Adlai Stevenson, claimed that several of his subjects, as well as he, were dominated by the expectations of their father or what they imagined them to be. Sometimes their need to please their father was so great that they had to bring him back to life in their imagination or dreams to try to satisfy it. Though not strictly comparable to Crane's experiences, they likely imagined how they hoped their fathers would respond someday to their accomplishments and then sought to realize them.

"If Kennedy's older brother Joe had lived, Jack Kennedy would have probably been teaching in the University today," William Manchester told me, "but he went into politics. It was difficult for him in the beginning. He was relatively shy and apologetic, but he gathered strength as he went along. The role of his father was enormously important. We all try to please our fathers, but Joe Kennedy was very difficult to please. In that sense he was the opposite of Churchill, whose father hated him. His father died when he was young. There's a very revealing piece that Churchill wrote late in life. It's called, 'The Dream,' in which he dreams his father comes back to life and confronts Winston. In the conversation in this dream, Winston does not once mention his successes.

"It's possible for me to identify with that because my father did not make very much of me or think I had much promise. He died when I was eighteen years old. He had lost his right arm in the Argonne in 1918. The second time I was wounded (on Okinawa) a Navy corpsman came up to treat me, and my first question was, 'Do I get a Purple Heart?' He said 'Yes,' and I thought of my father, and I thought, 'We're even.' Ever since then . . . I have now published eighteen books, which are translated in twenty-two languages and braille, and I'm still trying to prove myself to my father. But of course I can't do it, because he's not here. And I think that was a strong motivating force for Churchill. It's also true of MacArthur. MacArthur's father was a boy colonel in the Civil War. He won the Medal of Honor at eighteen. MacArthur was trying to improve that record and prove himself to his father.

"That's also true of H. L. Mencken. Mencken wanted to be a writer. He wanted to work for a newspaper. His father disapproved of that, and he wanted him to learn the cigar trade. That's what Mencken was doing when his father died. Again, I think he was either eighteen or nineteen. The day after his father's funeral, he appeared in the city room of the *Baltimore Herald* and said he wanted to work as a reporter. So there again you have the tie of his father. . . . I don't know of how many men that is true, but I think in men that have achieved a great deal, their memories of their fathers play a role."

"Do you see any of these people ever really coming to peace with themselves?" I asked. "Do any ever really feel that they pleased their father?"

"No. Not even Churchill. On one level he did, but on another level that anxiety was always there. Churchill was a depressive. I've been a depressive for forty years, and I think that the role of a father has much to do with that, too. I think if you want to live a peaceful, happy life, the best thing you can do is to be born of a father who is the town drunk. You're going to have no problems in improving his record. But if your father won the Congressional Medal of Honor and you are a soldier, or if your father was a brilliant member of the House of Commons and you're going into politics, then you're never going to be completely satisfied, because he will never be completely satisfied since he's dead and can't know what you're doing."

Of course, it's possible to interpret accounts of this sort in different ways. It's customary to view them prospectively and say that these people are responding to the dictates of unconscious conflicts or motives. They still exert choice and shape their own futures. But you also can view their lives retrospectively, arguing that their father's expectations, which were written on their minds from an early age, became their own aspirations, and they pursued them throughout their lives, much as Stephen Crane pursued the objects of his fiction.

What this suggests is that you often live out in your imagination many of the experiences you later seek, but in a less dramatic fashion than Crane. You imagine what your first date or sex encounters will be like, relying on the stories of friends or accounts you read about in magazines or novels. You imagine how colleagues and friends will respond to you if you win some prestigious award, and then spend your life pursuing it. You imagine long in advance the kind of home you want and the lifestyle you wish to lead, and then work toward achieving it. You may not have actually written out parts of your own life-to-be, as Crane did, but you already know much of it in advance, years before you live it. It may be stretching matters a bit, and we may be quibbling over semantics, but it's possible to construe this as living portions of your life in reverse.

Your ability to live your life on separate biological and experiential time tracks—your lived doubleness—has important implications for how you inter-

pret your life. Generally, the biographical format used to portray your life dictates that you order the events chronologically from birth through death. This
time-bound, lock-step format causes you to order many personal experiences
along a temporal continuum that may not apply. If you grant any reality to your
experienced life, then you have to entertain the possibility that this artificial way
of depicting yourself may distort who you are.

In her book, *Telling Women's Lives: The New Biography*, Linda Wagner-Martin, one of the biographers I interviewed for this book, offers an interesting perspective about the framework within which biographers seek to understand
women. According to Wagner-Martin, men's lives are mainly focused outward,
and the important facts of their life are external and public. Biographies of males,
therefore, mainly have been uncomplicated presentations of the persona, shaped
in the pattern of a personal success story. In contrast, the lives of women, which
represent a tightly woven mesh of public and private events—the monotony of
daily routines, mundane household chores, finding suitable outlets for personal
expression, the peacemaker role, meeting the needs of the family—often don't
lend themselves so easily to this linear formula. Because of this, biographies of
women have failed to take into account the nonlinear nature of their existence
and the often hidden drama in their interior lives.

I'm not sure I agree with this distinction between the sexes, but I do agree
that any fuller understanding of people must take into account the interwoven
nature of their inner and external lives. When that happens, you find that the
time dimension you live in is arbitrarily imposed on you by biological considerations and convention and often doesn't reflect how you experience your life.
Stephen Crane's peculiar experiences illustrate how people can live a future event
in their imaginations before it happens. They also reveal how the plasticity of
your imagination lets you defy the biological linearity of time.

Some years ago I examined a middle-aged man who had some unusual com-
plaints. Increasingly and for longer durations of time, over a five year period, he
was bothered by strong feelings of knowing people he didn't know and having
been in new places he never had seen before. At other times, he had the opposite
sort of spells. Many people he knew well seemed strange to him and familiar
places seemed unfamiliar. These disorienting feelings were becoming more incapacitating at work and in his social life because he feared saying or doing something embarrassing. Growing more doubtful about the validity of his experi-

ences—"Do I really know this person?" "Have I been here before?—he began doubting his sanity and wondering if he was having a nervous breakdown.

These *déjà vu* and *jamais vu* experiences, which were later diagnosed as being caused by a cerebral aneurysm near his temporal lobe, raise some important questions about the reality of time and the nature of personal experience. When under the influence of a *déjà vu* experience, this gentleman essentially lost his sense of the present, which he now perceived as the past. Biologically, he moved forward in time, but experientially, he felt that he encountered all these new events before. These spells contrasted dramatically with his *jamais vu* experiences, in which he responded to his past experiences and recollections as he might toward happenings in his present and future. Although he recognized people and settings, they seemed alien and strange, as though he was experiencing them for the first time.

What this shows is the importance of intact brain functioning for your sense of past, present, and future. To correctly place an event or experience along a temporal continuum, you rely not only on your memory, which happened to be normal in this person, but on an emotional response to this event or experience that lets you know if it's familiar or not. Though oversimplifying a complex matter, I suspect that the neurophysiological orienting response, which lets you focus your attention on potentially important stimuli, may contribute to your sense of chronology. When you encounter novel events, you ordinarily experience some degree of emotional arousal. With multiple exposures to these same events, this orienting response, along with its associated sense of newness, gradually disappears. This habituation to new events likely contributes to your sense of familiarity.

You can find many instances among humans where experiential time and biological time don't seem to be moving in similar directions or at the same pace. As your ability to learn and retain new information progressively decreases with age, your attention moves more and more to those past memories that are firmly embedded in your mind, sometimes making your past more salient than your future. Nor is brain pathology always indispensable for these distortions in time. People exposed to traumatic events when younger may continue to experience them again with the same compelling, hallucinatory vividness during spontaneous flashbacks or after triggering stimuli. Individuals with multiple personalities appear to exist in a time warp and wreak havoc with all conventional notions of time, having various persona fixated at different ages, with one or another becoming prominent at different times.

The reason that the gentleman with these different "*vu*" experiences found them so debilitating was because he was losing his temporal moorings and couldn't trust his senses any longer. When everything seems familiar, as happens with *déjà vu*, there can be no sense of future. When everything seems strange, as happens with *jamais vu*, there can be no past. Losing confidence in his ability to place events and experiences correctly in time, he experienced his self as collapsing. With good reason. Without being able to arrange his experiences along a temporal continuum, he couldn't assimilate them into his ongoing life story.

THE STORY THAT IS NOT A STORY

Because a personal life story is so important for your sense of self, let me recap its essential elements. One of these elements is that you be able to consciously experience progressive change in your life. Your developmental unfolding insures that you become aware of the passage of time and your relative position along the life cycle. Narrative flow, almost by definition, depends on direction and movement. The second element of a personal story is that you can distinguish yourself from others. Without the presence of another human being, you have no way to define yourself. In a solipsistic universe, a single self becomes the equivalent of all people or merely the expression of God.

To emphasize these points, let me retell the biblical story of Eden to show that it's mostly no story at all, and only becomes a real story when these two elements are present. To this end, I'll assume that the biblical account of the creation story in the Garden of Eden is literally true.

In the beginning, the Lord God creates the heavens and the earth and all living creatures. Then He forms man from the dust of the ground, breathes life into his nostrils, and puts him smack in the Garden of Eden to tend it. He tells man that he may eat freely of every tree that is pleasant to sight and good for food, except for the Tree of Knowledge of Good and Evil, which stands in the middle of the Garden. If man disobeys this warning, he will lose his innocence and experience death.

So here is Adam, without care or want, wandering endlessly and aimlessly about, plucking delectable fruits off trees and biting into their fleshy pulps or spitting out seeds, perhaps also taking pleasure in his own body, with no other ambition than to "be." He has no need for language since there is no one for him to communicate with. He has no social role since there is no society. He has no conflicts or aspirations since all his needs are met. He is without guile or cunning since these qualities have no use. He has no need to succeed or compete since he already is first in the eyes of God. He has no need for knowledge since this will detract from his innocence. Besides, there are no books, music, or art available anyway, so intellectual curiosity will do him no good. He has no sense of self since he is the only one who exists. He has no personal life story since he leads a life without variety, without change, and without plot—with no beginning, no middle, no end. He has eternal life and Paradise, an existence without need, pain, or conflict. What more can he ask? Yet inexplicably, as days follow days, years follow years, centuries follow centuries, for eternity, he experiences a growing boredom and discontent.

Then the Lord God, in His wisdom, decides that it's not good for Adam to be alone and, after causing him to fall into a deep slumber, makes a helpmate for him out of one of his ribs, a being known as "woman" because she is part of "man." It's at this point that Adam gets the first glimmerings of a sense of personal self, as he begins to communicate with Eve, but his self-ness is negligible since she remains subject to him and he still has no wants. In the development of a personal identity, Eve, though, is more advanced, for she already has a rebellious spirit and constantly urges Adam to eat of the forbidden fruit.

Eventually, he succumbs. It's only after the Fall, when they both are cast out of the Garden of Eden and beget the long line of the begats and begottens, that Adam and Eve become mortal and the personal stories of man and woman begin. Only then does each begin to exist in time and space. Each enters a personal life cycle and now must distinguish between the sense of "I" and the sense of "we."

While you may continue to dream of recapturing that idyllic time before the Fall—that undifferentiated, mindless, care-free, womb-like existence, which your progenitors, Adam and Eve, lost—it remains unattainable as long as you retain a personal sense of self. Paradise happens to be a place where time is nonexistent. Without time, you can have no new experiences. Without new experiences, you can't live out a personal life story. Without having a personal life story, you can have no sense of self.

"Do you believe in Crane's case there was a good deal of illusion, a public persona to get beyond?" I asked Christopher Benfey.

"Sure, I think there are all kinds of masks and false fronts that Crane assumes. . . . But I'm a little uncomfortable with the too easy distinction between a false front or public self on the one hand versus the real self or the authentic self on the other. I think especially for a writer like Crane, that distinction was not always entirely clear for him, and much of what a writer does is to put forth imaginative other selves. They tend to take on a reality that his original self doesn't have for him. When Crane keeps saying, 'I cannot help disappearing and vanishing, it is my form of trait,' that seems to me a very common feeling that an artist may have. It's what Keats called 'negative capability.' The artist, when he or she is most involved in the creation of art, has a sense of disappearing, of vanishing, of losing or scooping out whatever original sense of self he or she had and projecting an imaginative self that has a fuller reality."

COMPOSING A LIFE

Whether you believe that you have the power to shape your own life or are fated to do what you do, you can't help construing your life within a story format. There are many reasons for this, but the most important, in my opinion, is that you rely on stories to give coherence to your sense of self and make sense out of your existence. Your personal life story offers you an opportunity to integrate in a cohesive and understandable way the seemingly immiscible mixture of your many biological urges, psychological needs, social responses, and spiritual yearnings. Without some organizing framework for these often competing and contradictory experiences, you likely would be emotionally incapacitated.

Since I rely on a narrative framework to explain many aspects of human behavior, I need to clarify what such terms as "life," "story," "role," and "script" mean. As a general guide, consider that you are born into a life and live out a story in which you adopt certain roles requiring certain scripts. In this process of becoming progressively differentiated from others, you may experience incompatibilities at the different interfaces. Your personal story may be unsuitable for the life you are born to or it may allow the full flowering of your potential.

Your roles may fit or not fit your personal story. And the scripts you employ may be inconsistent with your roles or let you function successfully in them. Let me elaborate.

BEING BORN INTO A LIFE

At the start, much like Adam, you are born into a life. You enter the world as a human being, a biological organism, with potentialities that may or may not be realized, depending on the influences to which you are exposed. Your life itself has no form or meaning as yet, other than the necessity of it being lived. The general parameters of your life are the same for all other members of your species. You progress from inception, to birth, to childhood, to adulthood, to old age, and to death, revealing all the properties of living forms. To live a life, all you need do is to eat, sleep, procreate, protect your territory, age, and fulfill your biological destiny. You don't necessarily need to be conscious of who you are and what you do and why you do it. Mostly, you live your life oblivious to the many forces impinging on you that determine what you can or can't do—your genetic makeup, your biological constitution, the neurophysiological workings of your brain, climatic conditions, the availability of natural resources, familial, social, and cultural programming, historical forces, and other unknown factors. Much of the time, you live your life instinctively as part of the animal kingdom, especially during infancy and childhood—the age of innocence—without seeking meaning in what you do.

ENTERING A PERSONAL STORY

With consciousness, reflection, and a sense of time, you enter your personal story. A personal story requires that you possess a self that can serve as a protagonist, someone who can act on the environment and be acted upon by it. Mostly, the broad outlines of your life story are already set out for you at birth and during childhood by the life you enter, as dictated by your biological makeup, family background and cultural heritage.[2] These early influences usually decide the kinds of people you're drawn to, the appeal of certain occupations, and the lifestyle you pursue.[3]

As part of a life story, other characters must exist as well. You aren't an island unto yourself, even when you try to be. You are reared by parents, compete with siblings and peers, work for superiors, select mates, and encounter adversaries. Because you are a social creature, you rarely have the luxury of carrying out your own plot without it impinging on others' lives. You not only inhabit other people's stories, but they also inhabit yours. More likely than not, frictions will develop between you and others, obliging you to modify your story plot. However, if your story-line happens to be important enough to you, you stubbornly cling to it, even if that involves upsetting others.

Whatever your personal story, you must live it in a cultural context. One of the major functions of cultures is to insure a cohesiveness among its members through common languages, codes of behavior, customs, rituals and belief systems. Each culture has its own mythology containing the common dreams and aspirations of its collective people. It's from this vast reservoir of mythic offerings, which are filled with struggles between heroes and villains, good and evil, and the quest for everlasting life, that you derive your own personal story. Myths of this sort serve as harmonizing and stabilizing forces that integrate people with their societies and nature.[4]

Even though your cultural mythology supplies you with the major elements and themes for your personal story, the story you eventually enter isn't always clearly articulated. Stories can be coherent or incoherent, cohesive or fragmented, developed or undeveloped, or rich or poor in content. They also can have different narrative tones, some being upbeat or credulous, others being downbeat or cynical. Not all people embark on a cohesive and developed life tale. Perhaps in the past, when people's livelihoods, social status, educational prospects, and future opportunities were mostly determined at birth, you could predict the course of their lives even before they set forth in the world. With the dissolution of the family, scientific challenges to established beliefs, rapid political change, and shifts in values and attitudes, the similarity and stability of many personal stories begin to disappear. In industrialized, wealthy societies, new stories proliferate and offer a broader range of options.

Just as every personal life story has a protagonist, it also has a plot. And a plot or story line represents an unfolding goal or purpose—the quest for immortality, power, control, knowledge, security, or pleasure—that follows a temporal course with a beginning, middle, and end. Even if you somehow manage to lead a relatively conflict-free or uneventful existence in a controlled, regulated environment, as Adam originally did in Paradise, your exposure to the passage of time itself creates a plot since with each succeeding day you change and are one day closer to death.

Naturally, your circumstances and personal inclinations shape the range of stories available to you. The more coherent and cohesive the story, the more it reconciles all the discrepancies and loose ends in your life, the more relentless and attractive its pull, the more each chapter inexorably follows another. You may be drawn, for instance, to the typical middle-class story of professional success, a home in suburbia, membership in a country club, church affiliation, and social respectability. Or you can live out a story for musicians and singers from the 1960s, a frenetic, driven life of alcohol, drugs, outrageousness, and social protest, culminating in your own self-destruction, a story played out so well by Jim Morrison, Jimi Hendrix, and Janis Joplin—a story also well known to Kurt Cobain, of the group Nirvana, who also followed suit—all of whom managed to kill themselves at the same age of twenty-seven. Or you can enter the typical life of a daughter of an alcoholic father and a long-suffering mother, by marrying an alcoholic husband, divorcing him because of his drinking, marrying another alcoholic, or perhaps for variety a cocaine user, and then raising alcoholic or drug-using sons and unhappy, caretaking daughters. Or, whether talented or not, you can lead the unconventional life of an artist or poet, nursing your angst and wrestling over the meaning of life in ateliers or cafes. Or you can live out the predictable life of the chronically unhappy housewife, bored by your life, resentful of your husband's perceived freedom and control, wanting to do something meaningful, yet too scared to strike out on your own. Or you can live the life of a high-roller, full of excitement and adventure, sports and gambling, exploring new experiences and living on the edge. Or you can enter the world of high society, associating with others of similar backgrounds and engaging in all those activities that go with your social rank. The stories go on. There is even one if you find none suitable. You can go about reinventing yourself, cultivating eccentricities, saying and doing outrageous things, fabricating your past, and being the center of attention.

Usually, one dominant plot subsumes several different subplots or themes. A major theme running through your life may be to fulfill your role as a parent or a spouse, or as the dutiful son or daughter to your parents. Another may be to serve God, your church, and community. Another may be to be successful in your career. All these themes represent only components of your basic story plot, which may be to lead an exemplary, traditional life as a guarantee for personal fulfillment and happiness. Or your dominant story plot may be the quest for power and success, with all else—family life, friendships, and recreational pursuits—representing only minor themes.

And on it goes. You become an active conspirator in your own life story. You move forward in your life by expressing your past and becoming the character you're biologically, psychologically, and socially disposed to be, if events and others let you.

Although the particular plot you live seems new at the time you're living it, others likely have lived it many times before, with minor details left for you to fill in or alter. As with fiction, original plots are rare. Most tend to be formula-driven and even hackneyed, especially the best-sellers. There's good reason for this. You tend to be drawn to conventional, ready-made plots because those are what your parents, teachers, and society trained you to prefer. Because most of the major parameters of these traditional plots are already implicit or spelled out, you never have to worry about losing your personal bearings, as sometimes happens when you embark on an unexplored course. But with whatever story you enter, you need to convince yourself that you potentially have some measure of control over its course. Unless you have your personal story imposed on you by force, accident, or circumstance, it enhances your sense of selfhood to believe that you select your own story, and not, as may be the case, that the story selects you.

It's important to note that your personal story doesn't only include what is actively transpiring in your life; it also corresponds to what you expect your life to be. You may live your life in obscurity, for example, yet constantly yearn for fame. Under ideal circumstances, your life story and basic aspirations coincide. When they don't, you keep working to reconcile them. If unsuccessful, you remain discontented and ill-at-ease unless you finally become resigned to your lot.

Because the story plot you follow offers a structure for your life, a vehicle for integrating your experiences, and a conceptual map to guide your way, you cling to it to keep from becoming disoriented. It becomes a *de facto* extension of you, familiar experiential territory for your life, and creates the context for your existence. This is why you try to preserve it at all costs. You may not play the prime role in composing your own personal life story, but you play a decisive one in safeguarding it.[5]

PLAYING ROLES

Within each story, you adopt roles, some of which are suited to your ends and others not.[6] A general story theme potentially may be realized through the adoption of assorted roles. For instance, if your main agenda is wealth and power, then you can pursue it through different routes—as a banker, a physician, a professional athlete, a politician, or vicariously through marriage. This is so for most of what you do, whether it be to live in the limelight, to be loved and admired, to lead an artistic and creative life, or to attack and confront authority.

Roles represent implicit or explicit expectations for behavior. They have evolved in society to meet various social needs and to reduce friction among people. Roles govern almost every aspect of social life. There are parental roles, sick roles, gender roles, professional roles, and leadership roles, for example, each defining appropriate attitudes and actions. Conflicts arise between people when their different roles overlap or their boundaries become ambiguous. Turf battles, animosities, and misunderstandings tend to be the inevitable consequences of role diffusion.

While you bring to your roles certain special personal features, they also exert powerful molding effects on you. They have a stability and momentum of their own, giving continuity to your identity, consistency to your actions, and constancy to your life, and enabling you, if they are suitable, to move more smoothly through your personal life story. For other people, the roles you assume convey important information about you and let them know what to expect from you.

Roles also serve as a basis for constructing your own personal identity. Because certain roles convey certain meanings in society, you can use them to represent who you are and base your self-esteem on how successfully you fulfill them. Although certain self-help approaches urge you to step outside your roles to find your true self, the roles you play actually may help you to feel more whole and coherent. Peter Sellers, the actor, articulated this well when he observed, "When my role is finished, I experience a sudden loss of identity."[7]

While the impact of roles on personal identity may seem more dramatic in many actors, that simply may be because you use less obvious stages. In his biography of Sir Laurence Olivier, Donald Spoto commented that in the striving for the widest variety of identities, Olivier ran the risk of being no one. Part of his attraction for stage roles seemed motivated by a self-loathing and dislike of himself. "I'm not a nice person," he claimed, "I can't wait to be this other person for three hours," referring to his time on stage.[8] Later in life he confessed that he often had difficulty in telling when he was and wasn't acting, or put more bluntly, when he was lying and when he wasn't. What solved this dilemma was for him to play an assigned part. "I suppose I am liberated only when acting," he admitted.[9]

During my interview with Donald Spoto, I asked him about the implications of his intriguing observation that after Sir Laurence Olivier's long, painful bout with dermatomyositis, he was able to be himself, whereas prior to that time he was mostly involved in roles.

"To be one's self, in the context in which I mentioned with Olivier, simply means to close the gap between who one claims to be in a celebrity famished society and who one was in the process of becoming. It's very important to tell you that I don't believe that personality is self, that identity is this static given, which someone has at birth and grows up to. It is a reality in process. . . ."

"With reference to Olivier, you made the statement, 'He was most himself when he was pretending to be another.' I think that's a profound statement, but you didn't clarify it in your book."

"The deepest sense that Olivier had of his talent, of his position in the world, of his position in English society, the deepest sense that he was getting at the truth of himself, was in his role playing. In this regard, a great creative person like Olivier was not just an actor but also a director and producer and a visionary of the theater and of film. Truthful role playing, when the actor submerges himself in a role and allows the truth of a character within a play to emerge, is a way of arriving at the truth. For Olivier, he was most himself when the truth of the role found a harmony and a consonance in the depths of his own fragmentation and allowed truth to emerge."

"Prior to his illness in 1974 you said that his needs were expressed in his art, but after his recovery they were expressed in his life. How do you see that transition being made and why?"

"The fact is that [with his illness] he couldn't work. He was thrown back for some kind of mysterious journey within that allowed the truth about his own life to emerge without access to roles, so that the great lord of the theater, lionized all over the world, became essentially "Larry." He allowed himself for the first time to be touched. The irony was that being touched was extremely painful. It was something out of a Kafka novel. It wasn't that he created mechanisms to allow this to happen, . . . but destiny imposed upon him a terrifying, painful, and isolating illness, which his own courage met. From that courage, from that dignity, and from some mysterious mechanisms that allowed him to confront it, he was able to get in touch with a deeper reality in himself that time and effort and work had disallowed him over the years."

Spoto's observation that Olivier was able to get at the truth of himself through his role playing gives us an important clue about the relationship of roles to the nature of the self. Contrary to common opinion, when you play various roles you're not necessarily being artificial or phony. These roles let you accentuate different aspects of yourself. Just as Olivier let the truth of a character within a play emerge when he immersed himself in a role, you also rely on roles to get at the truth about yourself, assuming that if a role fits and suits you, it represents who you are, and if it doesn't, then it misrepresents you. For certain roles, when you have the requisite talent, disposition and inclination, you play them comfortably and with ease; when that's not the case, you feel awkward, uncomfortable and constrained, as though you're wearing ill-fitting clothes.

As guides for how to play various roles, you often rely on role models, either by directly observing their behavior or incorporating images of them within you.[10] These internal images that you accumulate over the years of parents, teachers, celebrities, or other inspiring persons sometimes remain distinct and identifiable, but mostly they fade and become absorbed and assimilated into your sense of who you are. They provide the blueprints for your thoughts and actions, and keep you from responding haphazardly when you encounter new situations.

USING SCRIPTS

For each of your many roles, you have available a number of ready-made, prepackaged scripts that let you function effectively, efficiently, and convincingly.[11] You dress in certain ways, decorate your office in certain ways, act in certain ways, and say certain things that are expected of you when you play your parts. The requirements of your various roles tend to be almost ceremonial, conventional, and ritualistic, allowing for automatic and instant exchanges with others to facilitate social discourse. To play the role of a friendly neighbor, you utter standard greetings, comment on the weather, and offer other chit-chat and pleasantries. As an enlightened parent, you try to do and say all the things that enlightened parents are supposed to. As a celebrity, you make the usual authoritative pronouncements, speak elliptically, or make outrageous statements to show that ordinary standards don't quite apply to you. If you are a politician, you remain vague and equivocal so as not to give offense. And so it goes.

The importance of scripts is that they let you function comfortably in your roles. They are the basis for ritual and convention. They represent automatic, acceptable responses for a variety of situations and usually tend to be stereotyped and predictable. They play a large part in etiquette and decorum, telling you how to act in various social interactions at work, at home, and with your family. You may have several scripts to chose from for a particular role, but in time the scripts you use and the roles you play become intertwined. There are even common scripts for people who play the role of people writing their own scripts, such as being openly promiscuous, saying or doing outrageous things, and being tactless or self-centered.

Of course, you have a certain degree of freedom to make planned or impromptu changes in the scripts available for your roles, adding a distinctive stamp of your own, but that doesn't detract from the basic similarities that continue to exist. There's usually good reason for this since without a certain standardization in scripts, your behavior loses credibility for others or becomes less expressive of your role. It's as though an implicit protocol governs what you do and say and how you appear. Certain behaviors are associated with certain roles and others aren't. For example, you tolerate preaching from your preacher and not from your barber. "Feminine" women aren't supposed to be aggressive or outspoken. Employees are supposed to be deferential toward their employers.

The scripts represent a shorthand for informing others about your roles, and your roles represent a shorthand for telling them about the plots you've selected and the stories you're living. Scripts that are incongruous or inappropriate raise suspicion and gain undue attention. There's some slack about how you play your roles, but if you digress too much or are too deviant or too unorthodox, you can expect to encounter public censure or rejection.

PLAYWRIGHT OR ACTOR?

So powerful influences shape the nature and direction of your life, inducing you to inhabit standard life stories that have a beginning, middle, and end, and that mostly conform to certain culturally acceptable themes. Depending on your perspective, you can make a case for living your life prospectively, interpreting your experiences as the result of prior causes or personal choices. Or you can make a case for living your life retrospectively, interpreting your experiences as echoes of similar lives already lived or as already written parts you must play. Not unlike a Greek play, you act as though you can modify your fate, while the chorus of the voices in the background proclaims what you must do.

Whatever your perspective about causality, what transpires in your life needn't be as inexorable as it first seems. Playing a role and participating in a personal story aren't incompatible with personal freedom. To observe that Stephen Crane later led a life already conceived in his imagination is perhaps less amazing than the fact that he conceived of these events in the first place. Where did his phenomenal understanding of war or life with a prostitute or the nature of a shipwreck come from? There was no *Red Badge of Courage* or *Maggie* before he wrote them. These works seem to have been a product of his creative imagination, which brought into being something that didn't exist before. Therefore, if you say that he led his life backwards in time after his writing, you also must conclude that he lived it forwards in time before. This suggests that within the context of his own personal story, he has shown authorial freedom himself. Semantics? Perhaps. But with important implications about the extent of your personal freedom.

Pursuing Shakespeare's metaphor of all the world being a stage, we find that participating in a play needn't mean performing in rote fashion, with no opportunity for spontaneity or creativity. Like an accomplished actor on stage, you presumably have the opportunity for improvisation at times and can interpret your roles and the meaning of the story in your own distinctive way. And like Stephen Crane, you may be able to create the future before you live it.

Whoever the Great Playwright happens to be who formulates your personal story, provides your roles, and writes your scripts, he, she, or it seems to have created a mystery that underlies every personal plot, which has to do with the extent to which you can compose your personal life story or are only an actor in the unfolding drama. Obviously, you have little personal control over much of what is already written out for you when you are born into a life. But you may have more leeway in the course it takes than it first seems. You may not be the main author or even a collaborator in the composing of your life—since if it was largely up to you, you likely would have written it differently (perhaps choosing a longer life span, the absence of disease, more talent, or greater intelligence)— but you realistically seem to be able to function as a biographer, shaping and revising the material you have responsibility for, to make your life more meaningful and improve the quality of the story. This little bit of biographical freedom lets you believe that you can make crucial decisions at major forks in the road, to take "the road less traveled," so to speak. And, as I hope to show, you may well have that option, as long as you act within the relative constraints of your many roles and don't wander too far from your unfolding story plot.

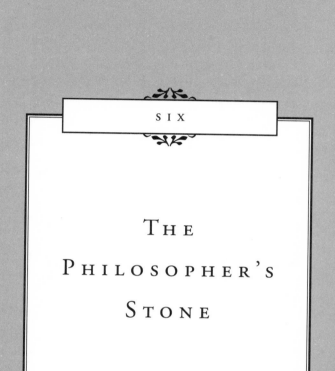

SIX

THE
PHILOSOPHER'S
STONE

ZOSIMUS OF PANOPOLIS, an alchemist who lived about 300 A.D., was the first to describe the existence of a philosopher's stone that could transmute "sick" metals, such as lead, into pure gold and also cure all human maladies. Since that time, countless alchemists throughout the ages have spent their lives searching for this miraculous stone. But in their futile quest to discover a substance that could change base metals into precious ones, they seem to have overlooked the possibility that this "stone-that-was-not-a-stone" was only a metaphor for one of the most remarkable gifts that humans already possess: the ability to transform bad experiences into good ones or to endow meaningless events with meaning.

As part of the human predicament, people endure pain, deprivation, beatings, rape, torture, imprisonment, exile, solitary confinement, insanity, humiliation, death of loved ones, terror, abasement, severe injury, debilitating illness, disfigurement, mayhem, starvation, betrayal, abandonment, sexual abuse, failing health, brain damage and other tribulations. It's remarkable enough that most of these people continue to cling so desperately to life, as miserable as it may be for them. What's even more remarkable is that substantial numbers of them manage to find meaning in their ordeal and also claim to be better for it. Some even believe themselves reborn.

Richard Pryor, the actor-comedian, admitted that he couldn't always control his arms because of multiple sclerosis. However, he wasn't complaining. "It's enabled me to deal with it up on stage, talk about it and make jokes about the hospitals and doctors. That's a gift," he said, "I didn't know it at the time but it's a gift."[1]

Ernest Byner, a running back for the Cleveland Browns, was about to score a touchdown that would give his team a chance to tie the Denver Broncos, 38–38, when he fumbled the ball. His team lost. As he looked back on the fumble, he opined, "It's like God had a plan for me. God had been trying to get into my life for a number of years, but maybe it took something to shake me into believing. That's what the play was all about."[2]

Several years after being diagnosed as HIV-positive, David Brudnoy, an author and talk-show host, wrote, "I live with AIDS realizing that the experience has not only been phenomenally instructive but also, oddly enough, enlightening, enriching, life-enhancing and liberating."[3]

Reynold Price's memoir offers another account of how someone can transform tragedy into triumph. After four years of surgery, radiation, medications, intractable pain, assorted humiliations and progressive paralysis caused by his spinal cancer, Price, a fiction writer, used his writing to emerge from his mental torpor. His early poems and later fiction were personal accounts of his affliction and how he tried to accommodate himself to his new life of pain and physical debility. With a resurgent sense of spirituality, he had a phenomenal increase in his creativity and productivity and became more compassionate toward others with misfortunes. He then claimed gratitude for the "whole new life" his suffering opened to him.[4]

This fortuitous adaptation to adversity can take many forms. A woman writer, experiencing excruciating pains in her back and leg because of a detached vertebra and the aftermath of surgery, came to view her illness as a metaphor for important aspects of her life. She interpreted the surgical effort to fuse her vertebrae as related to issues of union and detachment with her mother, her children, and her mate, and became concerned that her bones would not heal unless she could fuse her prior self with the woman she had become. Her illness, therefore, served to bridge the chasm between her physical and psychological being.[5]

As he accepted a check from donations to rebuild his church, which was destroyed by arson, Reggie White, an associate pastor and Green Bay Packer football star, said, "I always believe that out of something bad comes something good. I think God had a plan in all of it. I think this is a step forward in defeating racism."[6]

Accounts of this sort are endless. A woman interprets the sexual abuse she experienced during childhood as serving some higher purpose, because God never would allow a child to suffer as she did for no reason. A convicted political aide to the President has a religious awakening in prison, and then goes on to study for the ministry. A mother loses a child and contends that God has taken it. A soldier blinded by a head wound later credits his affliction for forcing him to develop his other senses and "see" what few others can see. Several years after a painful divorce, a woman says that she never could have developed confidence in her own abilities if she had remained in the marriage. In all these accounts, people encounter misfortunes, but instead of crumbling and calling it quits, find special meaning in what happened and inspiration for their future lives.

These accounts suggest that our basic inclination isn't to affirm the awfulness of our misfortunes, which often force us to make radical changes in our life story, but to keep from becoming demoralized by them. We're not only disposed to hold onto life until the last gasp, but to hold onto our basic assumptions about living as well. Our response tends to be more reflexive than deliberate in an attempt to preserve the integrity of our self.

As it happens, the self (a notion which, for now, will apply to all those mental operations that sustain our personal sense of being and identity) responds to traumas in much the same way as other bodily systems, such as the cardiovascular, musculoskeletal, endocrine, or immune systems do. Just as the natural response of a bone to a fracture or a muscle to a tear is to repair itself through the proliferation of new bone or muscle tissue, the self automatically responds to demoralizing predicaments, which potentially can cause rifts in its operation, by generating narrative segues and transitions between those predicaments and more favorable interpretations of them. Just as the natural response of the immune system to foreign bodies or germs is to manufacture antibodies or killer cells to destroy them, the self attempts to rid itself of any unwanted, incompatible, or unacceptable thoughts and feelings by denying responsibility for them or attributing them to others. Just as the natural response of the immune system is to wall off tissue damage caused by foreign bodies, resulting in abscesses when scarification of the lesion does not take place, the self often responds to massive psychological traumas, which it cannot discard, incorporate, or rationalize away, by walling them off from consciousness. Though imperfect, this compartmentalizing of noxious experiences is designed to let the self function without having these experiences contaminate its operations. Just as the natural response of the bodily defense system is to break down foreign bodies or dissolve blood clots that impede circulatory flow, the self often defends itself against threats to its integrity by deconstructing them. By decomposing these threats into their component parts and responding to each of these parts separately, independent of their overarching meaning, the self allows their significance in relation to the whole to disappear. As a result, deconstruction lets people justify anything they want to do. Only when all of these automatic mechanisms fail does the self go into emotional shock, much as the body goes into shock after acute blood loss or severe toxic reactions.

What we find, then, is that under normal conditions our self seeks to maintain the narrative flow of our personal life story. It does this by plugging unexpected leaks or mending any tears in the narrative structure with an assortment of sealing or bridging rationales. Much like a philosopher's stone, it can transform painful experiences that challenge our basic assumptions about the nature of our self and our reason for being into ones that are consistent with them.

AN ALCHEMIST'S BREW

Various cultural myths, often institutionalized by religion, help to shape our basic assumptions and generate meaning in our everyday lives. They represent compelling bundles of needs, values, yearnings, attitudes and aspirations, packaged in narrative or pictorial form, which organize and give meaning to personal experience. One of their most important functions is to integrate us with our society. They do this by striking a balance between our own personal interests and those of our society. The most enduring cultural myths are those that manage to strike a balance between these often conflicting interests.[7] Like an alchemist's brew, these myths cast a magical spell over us, giving us the power to create our own psychological reality. They let us transform unknowns into knowns and tell ourself what we're biologically and socially inclined to hear.[8]

MASTER OR MISTRESS OF OUR FATE

One of the most appealing myths we embrace is the notion that we have control over our own lives and can construct our own futures.[9] We convince ourself of this in many ways. To counter the relative puniness of our bodies, especially compared to certain other creatures, we may extol our physical prowess, endurance, and strength in athletic feats and competitions. To deny the hold that biological drives have over us, we may resort to self- abnegation, self-immolation, or mortification of the flesh, controlling our hunger and sexual desires, stoically trying to rise above our passions and other physical needs, or seeking out-of-body experiences to ally ourself with supernatural forces. To substantiate our personal appeal and influence, we may seek to conquer others, seduce them, manipulate them, or exert power over them. To demonstrate our control over Nature, we may turn to science or philosophy to unravel the mysteries of the universe. To create the illusion of permanence, we may try to accumulate wealth, acquire property, establish estates, or create works that will survive our death. To affirm our sense of free will and personal choice, we may seek to reinvent ourselves. When we reach the limits of our natural powers, perhaps the most powerful tactic we may use is prayer, in an effort to control God. By pleading, bargaining, inveigling, beseeching, supplicating, acting submissive, and humbling ourselves, we try to get the Almighty to do our bidding.

It serves no purpose to realize that these monuments we build to our personal efficacy are only sand castles, which will be washed away in time, or that much of the control we exert over our lives is illusory. Fortunately, the way our minds work keeps us from experiencing this kind of despair. Because our thoughts usually precede or accompany our actions and we often accomplish what we set out to do, we assume that we're causing our own behavior, not bothering to wonder what biological or environmental forces may have influenced our thoughts. As long as we can experience our selves as the source of our actions, we're apt to believe that we have substantial control over our lives.

Other aspects of our mental functioning fortify this belief. With every act, every thought, every feeling, moment by moment, we're presumably in the process of affirming the existence of our selves and our ability to influence events. We do this by storing our experiences in memory, thereby establishing ownership over them. This ability to transform personal experiences into memories gives us an artificial sense of control, since once they are inside us, we have a chance to rework and revise them so that they're more consistent with our life stories. While we're living our experiences, other people and events play an important role in influencing how they turn out to be. But once we deposit these experiences in our memory banks, they belong exclusively to us and we potentially have the only say in how we reprocess them.

Another way we can convince ourselves of our ability to control events is through reframing our personal experiences. Even when we're powerless over what happens to us, adopting satisfactory explanations, which are consistent with our underlying assumptions and expectations, creates the impression of personal control. The events may not be of our own making, but the very process of assimilating them into our personal life stories in a way that makes sense gives us a sense of mastery over them.

THE PURPOSE OF PURPOSE

We all seek a purpose in life: to aid humanity, to worship God, to promulgate the truth, to advance some important cause, to create beauty, to raise a family, to further evolution, or to fulfill some Divine intention. We need to believe that what we do is important and matters, or why do it? Even if we can't believe in a particular spiritual, social, or political system, even if we can't fathom any purpose to human existence, we're forced to act as if there is meaning.[10] Meaning conveys a sense of preciousness to our experiences. It helps us construct rather than deconstruct our lives. Our alternative is to give ourselves entirely over to hedonism or to become emotionally paralyzed by disillusionment.[11]

To retain a sense of purpose, we must believe in our specialness. This specialness may refer to our physical attributes, our talents, our family background, our acquisitions, our accomplishments, our personality, our children, our affiliations, our outlook, or our secret longings and thoughts.[12] Because of this specialness, we are apt to presume our precious self as being worthy of preservation for eternity.

Part of the reason we cling to a belief in our own specialness is that it seems intuitively true. After all, we are our most prized possession. We're really all we've got and can be sure about while we live. This narcissistic view has survival value. Because of our presumed specialness, we're more likely to look after ourselves, if we don't become too entranced by our own image.

It's often the case that innovators, creators, and leaders have an exalted view of themselves. General Douglas MacArthur exemplifies this feeling of specialness and self-confidence almost in caricature. According to

William Manchester, MacArthur was a real paradox, both noble and ignoble, inspiring and outrageous, the best and worst of men. He was an insufferable egotist, carrying the plumage of a flamingo, and could never admit to being in error. He was endowed with great personal charm, a will of iron, and a towering intellect. He also was very brave, winning over twenty medals, thirteen of them for heroism. He yearned for public adulation, yet he was disdainful of public opinion. He needed enemies the way others needed friends, and his actions guaranteed he would have them. Though he never went to church, he professed a belief in God and regarded himself as one of the world's two great defenders of Christendom, the other being the Pope. At the height of his career, he was so taken with himself that he began referring to himself in the third person. He also installed a fifteen-foot mirror behind his office chair in Washington to amplify his image.

I asked Manchester how someone like MacArthur or certain of his other subjects can sustain attitudes of this sort.

"I think that these men, like most men, have more than one level of awareness. They can be honest with themselves, but not all the time. In order to drive ahead with the self-confidence, which is needed, they have to block certain things off."

I didn't say so at the time, but one of the obvious bits of information they have to block from their awareness is that shortly they will be dead.

Of all the ingredients in the alchemist's brew, meaning is perhaps the most important. It's the basic stock for all the myths that pervade our life. We can endure pain and death as long as there is meaning to our torment and our demise makes a difference. Suffering stops the world and cries out for meaning.[13] In the absence of meaning, melancholia and agony bring our life story to an abrupt halt. "Concentrated is the soul," wrote Heine, the great German poet, "in the jaw tooth's aching hole." People can endure the worst abuse if they tell themselves it's for some higher purpose, such as for the sake of their children, to preserve their marriage, for the good of their country, or for the glory of God. Nietzsche claimed, "He who has a why to live for can bear with almost any how."[14] If nothing matters, then we have no incentive to do anything. In the absence of meaning, in a nihilistic universe, even suicide loses its appeal, since the act of taking our own life implies a value that life isn't worth living.[15] To avoid this bleak prospect, we keep searching for meaning. If we don't readily find it, then we deliberately manufacture it even when we know that it may be artificial and unreal.

In his play *Waiting for Godot*, Samuel Beckett showed how even in the face of an absurd existence, characters need to generate their own meaning.[16] Two of his characters spend their days contemplating suicide and engaging in twaddle, waiting to meet someone they don't know at a location they aren't sure about for some obscure purpose. As one of the characters says, "We'll hang ourselves tomorrow. Unless Godot comes." "And if he comes?" the other asks. "We'll be saved," the first responds. But Godot never comes, and they are never saved, and they continue living their lives and trying to keep their appointment every day with their would-be visitor just as they did before.

From his own experiences in a concentration camp, Victor Frankl, who based an entire system of psychotherapy on the search for meaning, found that if the inmates could find purpose in a setting that almost proclaimed the meaninglessness of existence, they were more likely to survive.[17] He describes, for example, how as a prisoner he found refuge from the emptiness, desolation, and spiritual poverty of his existence by escaping into the past. When given free rein, his imagination nostalgically played with past happenings, glorifying them and reaching out for them again longingly. By generating his own meaning, he was able to endure the privations, sufferings, and humiliations during this horrific time.

Much of people's daily existence is involved with mundane, humdrum pursuits that command low levels of meaning: housekeeping, work, recreation, sports, social life. Obsessives generate meaning for themselves through their ritualistic acts and endless repetitions. Even chronic mental patients find meaning in their day-to-day ward routines and the satisfaction of their creature comforts. They may look forward each day to queuing up at the nursing station to receive their daily medications or eating meals or going on a recreational outing. What sustains us is the meaning we impose on the activity and not the activity itself. Even when we do "nothing" but lie about, we're apt to justify this as a time for reflection, relaxation, or rest, assigning a purpose to the nonactivity.

One of the reasons that narrative is so important in construction of our life story is that language, by its symbolic nature, is designed to convey meaning. As poets, advertisers, preachers, and politicians well know, words represent condensed packages of information and, as such, carry meaning to people. When they are strung together in phrases, sentences, paragraphs, and stories, they gain in meaning. Any life story that moves forward in time generates an inherent meaning and implies an overarching design since there must be some reason for the juxtaposing and sequencing of experiences. Even in the process of mentally conversing with ourselves, we automatically imbue our thoughts with meaning because of the presumed purpose behind them.

LOVING THE BOND

Another way we try to guard ourself against the potential meaninglessness of existence and the finality of death is by believing that we matter to others. If we matter to others, then we suppose our selves to be important. Early on, those others are our parents and members in our immediate family. Later, those others are our teachers, our friends, our colleagues, members of our church, our employers, and if we are creative or make discoveries, our audiences and our public. Then, posthumously, if we become famous enough, those others are posterity, or if we aren't famous enough, an All-Knowing Being, who created us in His image.

As Peer Gynt eventually discovered, another's loving image of us gives constancy and substance to our self. The self can't be an illusion if others love it. They must be responding to something real, or so our philosopher's stone tells us. A friend informs me, "If I'm not loved, I don't exist—I'm nothing." If others love and need us, we reason, then we're vital to their existence, and being vital to their existence gives us a prominent place in the altar of their minds. It makes no difference that those who love us may be more in love with their image of us than with who we actually are. Our parents may love us as extensions of themselves and as the grown versions of the children they have known, never being privy to all the experiences, feelings, and thoughts we keep from them. Our children may love us as remote figures with exaggerated failings and strengths. And our mates or lovers may love us possessively, knowing us in ways that hold special meanings for them.

Why then does being loved matter so much when we know that others, because of their love, may be seeing us through distorted lenses or blinded to reality? I'm reminded of a woman I'd been seeing in therapy for several years. I was taken aback one day when she haltingly confessed her love for me. At the time, trying to put her admission in a more realistic perspective and feeling more threatened than I let on, I remembered saying, gently, "You mean you feel close to me because you can share personal matters and because I seem to understand."

"No, I love you," she persisted.

"But you can't love me. You hardly know me," I protested, not wanting to explore the mine field of issues her declaration might raise. "You don't know my beliefs, the books I read, my tastes, my hobbies, or my habits."

Exasperated, she countered, "You just don't understand."

It was only much later that I realized she was right. I really didn't understand her. Pathologizing her love as the result of unresolved Oedipal feelings was doing her a disservice. She did love me in her way, but her loving me had little to do with me, the presumed object of her love. But this didn't make her love any less real than the love of my spouse, my friends, my parents, or my children for me. They simply loved me in different roles, based their love on different categories of information about me, loved me according to their own needs, and loved me in different ways.

If these people know me incompletely or even inaccurately, can I take any solace in their love? Yes, but only if I can accept that they're in love with their image of me, and if their image of me changes, their love may no longer exist although I remain the same person. The games Puck played with his love potion in Shakespeare's *Midsummer Night's Dream,* causing unlikely characters to fall in love with one another, make this point well. Sometimes the "real" nature of the loved person can be irrelevant. The importance of being loved doesn't lie in being understood by those who love us but in the bond it forms with them. This bond affirms the illusion that we in particular matter to them, and because we do, can expect support and care from them while we live and being remembered by them after we die, even if the remembrance is only a distorted image of us.

From the vantage point of Nature, the attributes of the beloved seem less important than the love bond itself. This bond extends the personal boundaries of others and brings us under their protective umbrella, which also at times can seem like a prison. The bond exists as a way to link us together for the purposes of procreation, child-rearing, family solidarity, close friendships, and other special relationships. These emotional linkages help to reduce our sense of personal insignificance, keep us from facing the vast universe alone, and perpetuate our image in their memories.

During my interview with Scott Donaldson, he commented on the great desire of many fiction writers to be liked by others, and, as I construed his comments, their great need for love.

"I now have five biographies, and the first was about a very obscure American poet named Winfield Townly Scott. I really liked his poetry. He'd been a newspaperman, as I had been, and then there was this very close identification . . . because he was not a great writer. [He was] a very good writer, but someone that I could compare myself with and compete with intellectually. [Anyway,] I once saw in his journal a comment that he was out watering the lawn and there were some birds around and he tried to avoid spraying them, and he thinks to himself, "God, do I want even the birds to like me?" I see this in writers. This is the same [quality] Bill Clinton is being accused of as a kind of character flaw. He says nice things to everybody and wants to please everybody because he wants them to like him, and this is thought to be dangerous, and maybe it is. But I tend to see this quality in myself and in others. Not in Hemingway, but certainly in Fitzgerald and Cheever."

Now what about the other side of the equation? If being loved, liked, or respected helps to establish our link with others and affirms our selfhood, then so too should our caring about others. By loving others, we deny the potential meaninglessness of existence and add meaning to our own life. When others matter dearly to us, we want to be with them as much as possible, perhaps even for eternity. Every person we deeply care about increases our commitment to living and makes the prospects of our dying even more difficult to contemplate.

Since the bond established by loving or caring about others serves to ground our sense of self in the reality of their lives, it's puzzling why people stay in relationships that are degrading or demeaning to them, especially when they have other options available. How can people love others "too much," as the popular notion would have it, when those others abuse them physically, emotionally, sexually, or by neglect? How can people, for example, remain devoted to parents who treated them harshly as children? How can troops remain loyal to leaders who take them on suicidal missions and seem to have little concern about their lives? How can worshippers continue to humble themselves before a God who inflicts pain and suffering on their loved ones? These are critical questions that bear directly on this issue. The fact that many people do continue in these abusive relationships reveals something important about another dimension of love.

To make sense out of these abusive relationships, let's examine the common situation of women who supposedly love their abusive mates "too much," although there's ample evidence that something comparable can happen with men as well. Conventional wisdom has it that such protestations of love by these women are only face-saving excuses to remain in the relationship because they don't want to face the consequences of surviving financially on their own, dealing with their mate's anger or potential violence, facing loneliness, coping with the unknown, or worrying about what their parents and others will say. All of the practical and psychological reasons mentioned for staying married are important, but they don't seem to get at the root cause for this behavior. Some more elemental force, perhaps biologically determined, seems to be contributing to the power of this bond.

If so, what could this more elemental, biological force be? The results of recent studies suggest that there may be a hormonal basis for bonding or mating, at least in prairie voles.[18] Oxytocin and vasopressin, which are secreted in the brain during sexual arousal and intercourse, seem to cause bonding in sexual partners and make them inseparable until death. Oxytocin brings out the nurturing instinct in females, and vasopressin induces males to mate for life after one marathon sex encounter. They seem to function as internal love potions that cement the relationship, despite the particular qualities of the creatures involved. Although it seems reasonable to speculate that hormones such as these likewise underlie monogamous relationships among various animal species, no solid evidence exists yet about their role in humans. Even if these hormones were found to play a role in male and female bonding, what their presence wouldn't explain, though, is why males continue to abuse their partners. As it happens, once bonded, male voles actually treat their mates nicer than they treat other voles and become more helpful around the nest.

The more conventional way to explain dominance and submissiveness is by means of a social dominance hierarchy, which is prevalent throughout the animal kingdom.[19] For example, we know that within communities of chimpanzees, the alpha male looms above all others, strutting erect with his long hair standing on end and causing others to cower under his ferocity. We also know that when dominant male monkeys attack a female, she immediately assumes a submissive posture. Among chickens, cocks always dominate hens, so a breeding stock usually has separate pecking orders for each sex. Evidence also is mounting that these dominance hierarchies involve more than social behavior; they appear to have a hormonal or neurochemical basis.[20] An increase in androgen levels, which results in the masculinization of anatomical and behavioral traits, tends to move animals up the hierarchy. The adrenal hormones, such as 17-hydroxy-corticosteroids, 17-ketosteroids, and various neurotransmitters also have been implicated in social status.

With observations such as these, it does become possible to draw parallels between certain animal behaviors and the relationships sometimes noted between dominant and submissive persons. But a social dominance hierarchy also leaves much unexplained. We still are left with the paradox, for example, of women who continue to "love" their abusive mates even when they are out from under the yoke of the relationship, sometimes remarrying the same men after divorcing them, grieving for them after their deaths, or seeking out other men like them. Of course, there may be psychological reasons for this, but behavior of this sort may be biologically based as well. It was Mary Wollstonecraft, a pioneer in the women's suffrage movement, who in *A Vindication of the Rights of Women*, published in 1792, hinted at what this biological force might be. Attributing the wretched and weak status of women largely to a false education, she explained, "Gentleness, docility, and a spaniel-like affection are consistently recommended as the cardinal virtues of the [female] sex."[21] As it happens, her choice of words was remarkable. She described the relationship of many women to their husbands as similar to the slavish, emotional attachment a dog has for its master. And when she protested, "How grossly do [men] insult you who advise you to render ourselves gentle, domestic brutes,"[22] she seemed to be suggesting that the traditional dominion of women over domestic affairs may not be too far removed from domestication.

Could it be, then, that like certain species of animals—the cow, the goat, the pig, the horse, the sheep, and the dog—humans also are biologically capable of being domesticated? By "domesticated," I mean tractable, tame, socialized, obedient, compliant, and manipulatable. In the case of animals, this domestication is by humans; in the case of humans, by parents, authority figures, and certain leaders; and in the case of women, by men. In all cultures throughout history, aside from their poorer educations, limited freedoms, and lack of opportunities, women also may have been disadvantaged in competing physically with men because of lower androgen levels and less physical strength, and as a consequence, may have lacked confidence that they could compete and survive on their own. This likely contributed to their submissiveness to men. While domestication hadn't always been kind to women, their domesticity served a stabilizing social function, prompting a relatively selfless dedication on their part to the welfare of their children, their mates, and their homes.

Unfortunately, insufficient attention has been paid to the role that domestication may play in all kinds of social relations. To understand the nature of domestication, we need to understand the survival function it serves. Although the prerogatives of dominance include priority to food, water, and sexual partners, domestication also holds advantages for the domesticated species.[23] Evidence suggests that domesticated animals chose us as much as we chose them. Species capable of domestication drop their defense mechanisms for the tangible benefits of protection or food. The arrangement usually is mutually and evolutionary advantageous to both the domesticators and the domesticated when it results in a pooling of skills.

Neoteny, or the tendency to display juvenile features, is a common consequence of domestication.[24] As progressive generations of animals become domesticated, their adult behavior comes to resemble more and more the behavior and anatomical features their free-living ancestors displayed as adolescents. Like puppies, they're more likely to lick or fawn over familiar persons or display submissiveness and roll over on their backs.

Cartoonists have exploited the ability of neoteny to trigger biologically determined, innate releasing mechanisms for affection and nurturing in adult humans. Tracing the growing domestication of Mickey Mouse, S. J. Gould showed that cartoonists made him more lovable and less threatening by shortening his snout, increasing his eye size as a percentage of head length, and proportionately increasing the size of his head to his body: features associated with younger mice.[25] Donald Duck also underwent a similar transformation. These youthful features played on natural sympathies.

The parallels in humans seem too obvious to ignore. In many cases, domestication serves women's biological advantage: in exchange for their submissiveness, they often receive security from their mates, as well as the physical protection of their offspring. To insure this advantage, they display certain features associated with neoteny. As with the domesticated version of Mickey Mouse, especially in certain Western societies, they may emphasize the size of their eyes by using mascara, artificial eyelashes, and eyebrow pencils, and accentuate their mouths with lipstick. They may shave much of their bodily hair and try to keep their skin smooth and soft like babies. Cultivating deferential and vulnerable looks around men, they are more likely to elicit caring responses.

Men also may show comparable behaviors when they are in subordinate roles. The stooped posture, hunched shoulders, downward gaze, and docility shown by many men or, in certain cultures, their prostating themselves in the presence of superiors not only may resemble the responses of a submissive animal toward a dominant one but also the puerile responses of a domesticated animal toward its master. That also may explain why people in authority, such as military leaders, coaches or corporation executives, who interpret facial hair as a sign of independence, insist that male subordinates be clean-shaven, giving them a more youthful, smooth-cheeked, immature look.

Aside from the powerful demands of the dominance hierarchy on male-female interactions, it may well be, then, that women "who love too much" and remain in abusive relationships may not be masochistic personalities, as some psychiatrists claim, but are simply expressing a domesticated response to those wielding power over them. This response isn't so different from the respect and obedience adults may show toward domineering parents, the sometimes stupefying compliance of captives toward their captors, the deference and submissiveness of many slaves toward their masters, and the "identification-with-the-aggressor" responses of certain concentration camp prisoners toward their keepers. They've been trained to obey. They've been conditioned to be submissive and responsive to authority. They've been systematically broken and domesticated to comply with the wishes of those who wield the most power. Their compliant behaviors aren't simply motivated by fear, affection, or the desire for approval. They may partly behave as they do because of the powerful bond that becomes established between the domesticated and the domesticator, which those who become domesticated, for want of a better explanation, interpret to be love.

FOREVER AND EVER

All of the myths that we embrace largely stem from one fundamental concern. If we believe that we exert substantial control over our life, that what we do matters in the ultimate scheme of things, and that others truly love us, then it becomes difficult to accept the prospect of our nonexistence. We tell ourself that there must be more to life than death. We could not have been created only to be destroyed. But as a hedge against this disturbing possibility, we try to insure our survival in whatever ways we can, usually through our beliefs, our progeny, and our work.

In his powerful polemic *Denial of Death*, Ernest Becker argues that, other than acting on our biological urges, so much of what we do represents an attempt at terror-management.[26] We live our whole life with death hanging over us, like a Damoclean sword, while trying to deny our fate. Unable to reconcile the paradox of being able to contemplate the universe and still ending up as food for worms, we embrace beliefs that hold at bay our panic over dying.

Becker's arguments are cogent, but their emphasis is misplaced. It isn't death itself that we necessarily fear—many people risk their lives in daredevil feats, undertake dangerous missions, engage in perilous expeditions, sacrifice their lives for others, seek out martyr's deaths, or commit suicide. Rather, we fear the loss of our experiential world. When death can be seen as an opportunity for gain rather than loss, such as by advancing a cause, gaining martyrdom, joining loved ones, or doing God's bidding, it loses its power to evoke fear.

Also, in the natural course of events, if we don't die prematurely by accident or disease, our normal life cycle prepares us for our eventual nonexistence. As our world gradually shrinks with the loss of physical pleasures and mobility, and we lose our sight, hearing, and smell, as we abandon our life work, as friends and beloved family members die, and as our memories begin to fade, we are gradually being desensitized to our inevitable nonexistence. We even may come to welcome death when we no longer have much of a self to lose. Our fundamental fear, then, is not the cessation of life that comes at the end of a full life cycle, when our life story is essentially over, but the prospect of prematurely ending our life story when we have more chapters of living left.

As long as we remain in full possession of our mental faculties and are not too physically ill, we keep seeking out ways for some form of existence beyond death. Through procreation, creative works, good deeds, or involvement in some grand cause, we hope to lay our gravestone in the minds of others and have our legacies represent us. Sometimes our desire for immortality can be so powerful that, paradoxically, it may pose a threat to our lives. For instance, years ago, after a long Sunday drive, my wife, child, and I came back to a flaming home. Instinctively, not heeding the pleas of my wife, I burst into my smoke-filled study to rescue the manuscript I was working on at the time. Coughing and woozy, I just managed to get outside when my study exploded in flame. Had I lingered for a few more moments, I certainly would have been killed. And for what? In my quest for fame and immortality, I unthinkingly almost sacrificed my life, and (what made it seem so futile) for a novel that really wasn't very good.

Risking my life for my manuscript is what most parents would do for their children, true believers would do for their faith, patriots would do for their country, and ideologues would do for their beliefs. While the preservation of life is basic, sometimes even more important is the desire to identify with something transcendent or to participate in an ongoing and lasting cultural drama, which offers the prospect of some form of existence beyond death or everlasting life.

Some people spend a lifetime seemingly erecting monuments to themselves through their creative works. Their works, in effect, become them, especially when they leave scanty personal information behind that informs us about their private concerns and motivations.

Bearing on this issue, I asked Donald Spoto, who spent many years studying the life and works of Alfred Hitchcock, why Hitchcock seemed so secretive. "He had no memoirs, no letters," I observed. "He deflected personal interviews. He forbade a biography about his life. What was that all about? What was he trying to hide?"

"I don't think it was so much him trying to hide something," Donald Spoto responded. "I believe that this was the quintessence of the Victorian, Edwardian, English burgher. That is to say, he had given every single thing about himself in this extraordinary array of fifty-three motion pictures, of which forty can certainly be counted among the great works of art in any genre in our century. Hitchcock did not come from an era where the artist or celebrity sat down and explained everything for the benefit of the public. We didn't help him make his films. He wasn't going to help us to understand them or himself. I don't think it was a question of him trying to hide. I think that he was an extremely shy man. Having known him personally, I can vouch for that. Extremely shy, and his entire life was lived within an envelope of enormous emotional pain and psychological struggle. That can be said for more real artists than not. In this regard, he was not exceptional. I believe that what he resented or tried to avoid was what he had seen so many others subjected to, and that was the shallow presentation of themselves. He had done his work. He had given us these films. There is his spiritual autobiography in these films. They are remarkable personal documents."

Though believing in some form of personal immortality represents a measure of our desperation, since we do so in defiance of all reason, we have little other choice. If there is no legacy of our existence either in the future or an afterlife— if our line of offspring dies out, if all our personal works are destroyed, if our gravestones are removed, if the causes we embrace no longer exist, and if all memory of us is lost—then for all practical purposes, our life will have been in vain, and our sense of self superfluous. With this the case, then everything we take for granted and believe in becomes meaningless. Understandably, we balk at this prospect.

WHY BELIEVE?

Now for the fundamental question. Since consciousness can exist without our believing in a personal self, why do we need to be able to believe in a self or, for that matter, any of these self-enhancing myths at all? What biological function does this believing serve? Why not just live our life, propagate, and die, fulfilling our biological destiny with no more self-consciousness or introspection than other animals and lower forms of life?

The answer, of course, is that we can have it no other way. Whether by cosmic accident or design, our brain is a problem-solving organ, oriented toward insuring our survival. During our lifetime, our mind is called upon to solve an impossible equation for which there are too many unknowns, either forcing it not to compute, or if it's to continue to function efficiently, to substitute fillers for the unknowns. That's where belief, myth, fiction, and faith come in; they help to eliminate the knowledge gap. As the Bible says, faith is the substance of things hoped for, the evidence of things unseen. Myth and metaphor offer substitutes for reality. Belief gives ignorance and mystery form, neither of which has survival value, and lets us act without continually having to wrestle futilely with the unknown. The self is so evanescent, abstruse, and intangible that it needs constant affirmation and buttressing. We'd find it difficult to function in society if we kept doubting the reality of our self or the meaning of our activities. The capacity to believe lets us get on with the process of living. If there is a biological basis for faith, animal analogues should exist as they do for most other human capacities, such as insight, problem-solving, or learning. As it happens, there may well be. A dog waits patiently for days or for weeks on end for its deceased master to come home. A horse tries to leap over a high hedge at the prompting of its rider without knowing what to expect on the other side. During a stampede, a herd of cattle blindly follows the leader. Though these examples may be explained in different ways, they bear resemblances to human faith. In all instances, the animals continue to act in ways that lack justifying proof or ignore evidence to the contrary.

Since beliefs, by their very nature, are unprovable, they need to be fueled by emotional conviction else, under scientific scrutiny, they can't stand on their own. The more metaphorical the beliefs, the more fervor necessary to sustain them. That's where the limbic system in the brain, especially the amygdala—the ancient part of our brain largely responsible for supplying emotional valences to our perceptions—comes in. It's this part of our brain, when stimulated by LSD, pot, or occasionally alcohol, which imbues our notions, experiences, and thoughts with a heightened sense of significance, sometimes of revelatory proportions. At times, this stimulation may produce attenuated "eureka" experiences, causing us to attribute false significance to inconsequential cues or thoughts. An ashtray can become a mystical symbol. A random sentence spoken over the radio can contain profound, hidden significance. A nonsensical thought can become a universal truth.

Let me illustrate an important point about the nature of beliefs by recounting something that happened to me during an LSD experience years ago when I was studying the effects of this drug.[27] Sometime during the height of the drug reaction, I remember experiencing an intense desire to urinate. Standing on rubbery legs and undergoing all kinds of Alice-in-Wonderland distortions of my body, I noticed a sign above the urinal. As I weighed the words on the sign, I suddenly realized their profound import. Here, right before my eyes, was the answer to the universe. No wonder all past philosophers overlooked it. It was obscured by its very obviousness. Thrilled by this startling revelation, I rushed out into the hallway to share this universal truth with my colleague, who was monitoring my reactions. Alarmed by my zeal, he must have thought I lost my mind. When I informed him of my discovery, he stared blankly at me for a moment, not fully comprehending, and then suddenly burst out laughing. I was shattered by his response but then realized that he, being a mere mortal, couldn't appreciate the earth-shaking implications of the sign's message: "Please Flush After Using!"

Experiences of this sort aren't only limited to hallucinogenic substances, such as LSD, mescaline, peyote, or psilocybin. They occur in response to a variety of substances that cause profound alterations in consciousness. William James, for instance, claimed that alcohol intoxication often makes things seem more "utterly utter."[28] The crucial point to be made is that the meaning we attribute to our perceptions may have little to do with *real* meaning. Whether affected by artificial or natural means, our brains have the capacity to generate the sense of conviction that shields our beliefs against any assaults by reason. This primal, neurophysiological sense of meaning stamps our beliefs with the unshakable imprimatur of truth. Most of our most cherished beliefs about the nature of our selves and the purpose of our lives may have no more inherent truth than the sign, "Please Flush After Using." But that is irrelevant. What matters is that we're able to believe they are true, and because of that, act on them.

Buttressed by the certitude of our convictions, we're now able to confront the very forces in the universe we feel powerless against. By believing in our personal control, the meaningfulness of our life, and the enduring nature of our self, we can diminish our sense of insignificance and the threat of our eventual extinction. If we believe in an omniscient Being who has a personal interest in us, this also lets us become an active participant in the running of the cosmic drama. We can exhort this all-powerful parental figure to do our bidding— entering our body during Holy Spirit possession, sanctifying us during Holy Communion, watching over our loved ones, or answering our prayers—or at least take our pleas under advisement. Our faith blunts the cruelty of having to exist in a hostile universe that eventually will claim our life and those of all who matter to us, no matter how important we think we are. Pain and suffering may stop the world, but believing that they serve some important purpose lets us get it going again. Without the capacity to believe in and sustain myths of this sort, we couldn't exist as well as we do—unless, of course, we happen to make a credo out of nonbelieving.

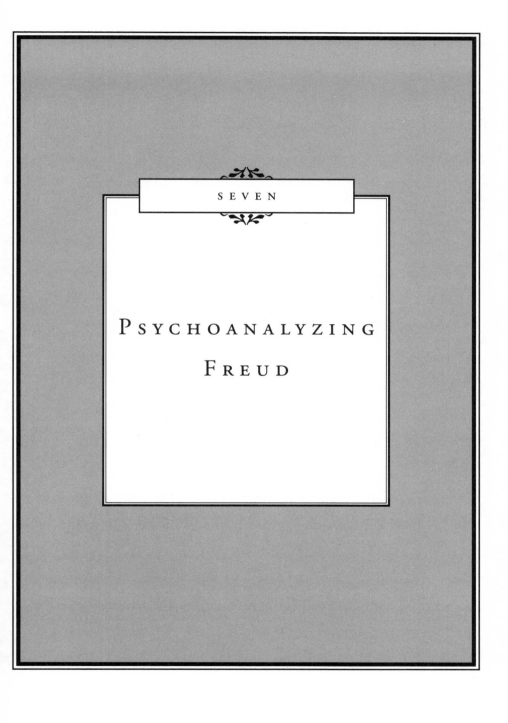

SEVEN

PSYCHOANALYZING

FREUD

YEARS AGO, when LSD was still being touted as a wonder drug, I experimented with using it as a form of therapy for drug addicts and alcoholics.[1] The results, at first, were astounding. Aside from experiencing wondrous colors and fantastic, panoramic visions, patients relived their pasts and had profound insights within relatively brief stretches of time, many claiming, as with a religious conversion, to be reborn and healed of their affliction.

"Now I understand why I got in so much trouble," exclaimed one, his eyes gleaming. "It was my old lady always hassling me, never giving me the benefit of the doubt. So I figured, if you're going to get blamed when you're innocent, you might as well have some fun."

"It was my father," complained another, the drug making the walls of the room pulsate for him with each beat of his heart. "The way he treated me . . . and the way he abused my mom. Whenever I think of that, I want to shoot up."

"I guess I've always had an inferiority complex," opined another. "My brother was the bright one, the successful one in the family, and he got all the attention. That's why I used drugs . . . so I wouldn't have to compete . . . and also to get back at my parents."

All of these insights seemed a little too pat, too face-saving, even though imbued with the conviction of divine revelation.

During revelations like these, each of these men glowed, certain that his insights would serve as springboards for a new life. Each experienced a spiritual conversion of sorts, a feeling of attenuated enlightenment, believing that he uncovered important facts about himself, which were responsible for his self-destructive behavior. There was only one problem. Their explanations, which remained suffused with the psychedelic conviction of truth, were no more effective in changing their attitudes and behaviors than the insights that other addicts and alcoholics gained from taking a placebo, such as a sugar pill. This raises the important issue of the relationship, if any, of psychological truth to objective truth.

VARIATIONS ON A THEME

For illustration, let's examine the famous case of Little Hans, which many credit as the start of child psychoanalysis.[2] By way of background, we should recall that Sigmund Freud invoked the Oedipus complex to explain the emotional problems of this five year old boy. Freud, who saw the boy only once, successfully treated him mainly by corresponding with his father. The boy's father, a physician himself, provided all the information upon which Freud based his interpretations and issued instructions for his treatment. Since this case represents a landmark in the evolution of psychoanalytic theory, we will resurrect it from the archives to examine how we establish the truth of any psychological interpretation. But this time we will add new wrinkles.

Imagine you're Hans . . . but "Big Hans" now, because it's twenty-five years later, and you have grown to be over six feet five inches tall. Unfortunately, you experience an embarrassing relapse of your old symptoms two weeks before you're scheduled to marry. As before, your symptoms include an intense fear of leaving your home—a problem that first began when you were a child, about nine months after the birth of your baby sister. But now, instead of your original phobia about being bitten by a horse, you dread being run over by a car.

Since you can't determine the psychotherapeutic orientation best suited for your problem, you replicate yourself so that you can undergo treatment simultaneously with famous therapists of different theoretical persuasions: psychoanalytic, Jungian, nondirective, existential, and cognitive-behavioral. After a course of treatment, you experience remarkable improvement despite the differences in theoretical orientation to which you are exposed. As far as you are concerned, your improvement confirms the separate truths of what each of your therapists told you about why you became ill. The dilemma for you, though, when you finally reintegrate yourself, is that each of your therapists espoused a different truth, some of which are mutually contradictory. Granting ourselves a license for exaggeration, let's recap what these different truths are.

The psychoanalyst continues to attribute your problem to castration anxiety as a result of an unresolved Oedipal complex, the threat coming from your anticipated marriage. When you were younger, if you recall, you were very close to your mother, wanting her all to yourself, but you feared that your father would punish you for this. When your sister was born without a penis—remember, as a child, you used to believe that everybody had a "widdler"—you saw what could happen to you if you didn't abandon your claim on your mother. So you identified with your feared father, symbolized in your unconscious as a huge horse with a huge penis. Now, as you prepare to marry your fiancée, who bears many resemblances to your mother, you experience a reawakening of the same unconscious conflict. Only this time, to modernize your symptoms, the horse, alias your father, takes on the form of a car.

Ignoring the realities of the moment, the Jungian analyst seeks the more mythic meaning, viewing your upcoming marriage as an important *rite de passage*, the transition from youth to adulthood. Within the collective unconscious, your reluctance to leave home symbolizes your insecurity about becoming independent and assuming adult responsibilities. The car, like the horse you once feared, represents a primitive archetype for all the external forces over which you have little control.

The Rogerian therapist refrains from offering an opinion about what is wrong with you because that will only compound the problem. It's your life, and what you want to do with it is up to you. If you're having anxiety about being hit by a car, perhaps you need to get in touch with what that anxiety is all about as you undertake the process of self-actualization.

The existential analyst interprets your upcoming marriage as an opportunity to confront your own being, to reconcile your personal inner world with that of humankind and the universe as a whole. The ancient problem is one of being versus existence. Unmarried, you sense your own incompleteness. Though you can become what you make of yourself, through your choices, you are unsure what you want. In the passage from nonauthentic to authentic existence, you have to suffer the ordeal of despair, facing the full implications of the limits of your existence—death and nothingness—before personal healing can take place.

Lastly, the cognitive-behavioral therapist views your anxieties and fears as the result of learned, irrational thoughts. At an early age, you learned to be frightened and timid because of your mother's overprotection and worries, and you continued that same pattern throughout your life. Since you can't undo the past, you need to correct your irrational thoughts and substitute more appropriate, rational cognitions for them.[3]

If you had happened to be born in other cultures, you would have been exposed to entirely different explanations for your symptoms. In Japan, for instance, because of the sacrosanct nature of the family, you would have romanticized and fictionalized the past, reinterpreting the actions of your parents as expressions of love, previously misinterpreted by you because of your immaturity. If you were brought up by non-Westernized parents in India, you likely would have attributed your emotional problems to evil spirits or to your karma from a previous life rather than to your psyche or personal history.

What this demonstrates is that there are many ways to account for the same phenomena, each purporting to be the truth, and all may be equally effective. What often makes a particular approach effective for you is for you to believe that it adequately explains your problems and offers you a way to deal with them. You can't expect a certain brand of psychotherapy to be equally suitable in all settings and for all people, like penicillin is for pneumonia, because different people harbor different perspectives of reality. If you happen to believe in witchcraft, for instance, you're more likely to be receptive to supernatural than to psychoanalytic explanations for your symptoms.

My introduction to the importance of the cultural context for therapy happened years ago during my training when I treated a seventeen-year-old Spanish-American girl, Maria, who, along with her mother and stepfather, was bewitched.[4] I admitted Maria to the hospital after her neighbors reported hearing blood-curdling screams coming from her house every night at midnight. Maria attributed her bewitchment to an event that happened at a family gathering in which her much feared aunt, reputed to be a bruja (witch), was present. During the evening, the aunt supposedly hypnotized Maria and forced her to have her hair cut, using it to make an effigy doll. Four nights later, Maria went into the first of her nightly trances. While in these trances, she would plead with the aunt not to throw her in cold water or to put the effigy doll in her grandmother's grave. On other occasions, she "took the baby's mind" and acted like an infant, or she would curse her mother, or would thrash about in the bed, as in labor, and scream out to the aunt, "You know I can't have a baby because I never mess around with anybody—you just want people to believe I'm pregnant." According to the parents, during one of her trances, Maria grew long fangs and nails and would scratch and revile them whenever they approached her. Her stepfather said that one of the best ways to bring her out of these trances was for him to jump on top of her to keep her from scratching him. Then he would throw his whole body on her and hold her tight and close to him for about ten minutes, after which she would come out of her trance.

The mother, along with her husband, held vigil at Maria's bedside every night. On the night of her first trance, they said that a huge black cat came into the kitchen after sundown, sat on the refrigerator and stared at them. They also noticed a pair of big red eyes in the window, watching everything they did. One evening, during one of her daughter's spells, the mother herself became bewitched, claiming to see a man dressed in black who told her that her husband and daughter were making love in the kitchen. There were two alarming occasions, according to the stepfather, when his wife, presumably in a spell, stalked him with a knife and shouted, "I knew something like that was going on between you and Maria. . . . You pay more attention to her than to me."

The stepfather also wasn't immune to these fearful happenings. Three times, while he and his wife were sitting by Maria's bed watching her while she slept, his wife noticed that he slowly began to rock back and forth and then gradually change into a yellow cat from the neck up. During these occasions, he himself became aware that his skin was getting tighter around his face and that when he tried to speak he would purr. On another occasion, while lying in bed with his wife, he happened to put his hand on her rotund belly, with its grapefruit-sized umbilical hernia, and was shocked to find that it turned into the flat belly of his step-daughter.

You don't have to be too psychologically sophisticated to guess about the underlying dynamics for this dramatic behavior. The witchcraft served as an ideal paradigm for this family to enact its conflicts without ever having to consciously confront the incest taboo. Since all were convinced the witch made them behave that way, no one was to blame for these terrible happenings.

The likely cause of Maria's behavior, which I suspected all along, was anathema to this family. The more I tried to lead them to an understanding of what was transpiring, the more I alienated them. At a loss over what to do, I turned to the local Catholic Church to enlist a priest who might be willing to undertake an exorcism. No such luck. This procedure was not to be taken lightly. Only specially trained priests could do this, and only after a decision had been made that the problem was indeed demoniacally induced. Since this wasn't a fruitful course to pursue, I then tracked down the bruja, hoping to convince her to give up the effigy doll. The aunt was an ugly, middle-aged woman with disheveled hair and crooked teeth, who fit the part of a witch. Though she admitted to cutting Maria's hair, she denied any knowledge of witchcraft. I then sought the aid of a curandera, a local healer, but to no avail. Eventually, I was forced to dissemble during therapy to resolve this refractory problem. Under hypnosis, I told Maria that I had taken the effigy doll from the bruja and that she was no longer under her spell. I also informed the parents that I had visited the bruja and told her to stop casting a spell on them. Within several days, Maria's trances ceased. As she got better, the mother became outwardly more assertive with her husband, and he seemed more cowed. Months went by after Maria's discharge, and I lost all touch with the family. One day, sometime later, the stepfather showed up in the hospital emergency room, shaken and distraught, and confessed that he had been having sex with his stepdaughter.

Not surprisingly, what this case shows is that there are different ways to interpret the same problem and that for a particular interpretation to work, it needs to conform to the world view of the person. For this family, the notion that the stepfather would initiate sex with his stepdaughter and that she would comply and that the mother would sense what was going on without intervening was incomprehensible. The obvious explanation for this unfortunate situation, one that would be acceptable and understandable to all, was that the witch was responsible. As long as I worked within that framework, even if it wasn't "true," the family remained receptive to my therapeutic interventions. Since belief in the witch let the family stay together as a unit, the family likely would have had to create her even if she didn't exist.

So, it seems that the way you come to understand yourself and deal with your symptoms depends, to a large extent, on your cultural background, on which therapist you happen to go to, on your therapeutic orientation, and how satisfied you are with the results. But because the different systems of psychotherapy yield much the same rates of success, provided that the therapists are of relatively equal skill, you find a puzzling situation in which there can be many different and often contradictory truths or one in which truth, as you know it, doesn't seem to matter.[5]

FREUD'S RECANTATION

Apocryphally, a key breakthrough in the development of psychoanalysis centered on this very issue of psychological truth.[6] Throughout the early 1890s, Freud believed that all cases of hysteria stemmed from sexual abuse by the father when the woman was a child. He claimed to have found evidence of this in seventeen of the eighteen cases he treated. Most of his professional colleagues greeted the formal presentation of his seduction theory for hysteria with disbelief and hostility. Despite the progressive drop-off in patient referrals, he continued to believe the lurid accounts of his patients until the later 1890s when his doubts began to grow. These doubts were partly prompted by practical considerations—he couldn't complete any of his therapy cases since offended patients left him part way through their analyses or didn't respond as they should. He was also partly prompted by reason—with hysteria so widespread in Victorian society, he found it increasingly difficult to implicate so many fathers, especially when not all victims of sexual abuse fell prey to hysteria. This led him to the conclusion that it was difficult to tell whether the sexual abuse actually happened or was imagined by patients since unconscious memories were so susceptible to distortion. His doubts about his seduction theory demoralized Freud immensely but eventually led him to an important clinical insight: the fantasy could be as important as the reality, and, for all practical purposes, represented psychological truth.

This presumed equivalency of fantasy and reality was hailed as an important milestone in the development of psychoanalytic theory. It freed therapists from the necessity of establishing the objective truth about what patients reported. The important fact was that they reported being abused and believed it. So far, so good. But Freud may have not gone far enough in his assessment. He didn't thoroughly examine his own motives for abandoning his original contention that most of the claims of early seduction were, indeed, true. Had he done so, he not only might have forced the medical profession and public to recognize how widespread the sexual abuse of children really was but also documented its devastating impact on the victims years sooner than this information became known.

But as Freud has taught us, the obvious reasons aren't always the real ones. Sometimes they serve to mislead the observer. The mystery is what led Freud, an astute clinician, to recant his seduction theory after stubbornly defending it for many years against the ridicule by colleagues. Since his reasons for doing so lie at the heart of what is psychological truth, we should be wary of embracing the convenient explanations he gave. Other reasons are possible. In the past, various authors have speculated that he did so to protect his own father or because he was having an affair with his sister-in-law or simply because of his failure of moral courage.[7] Any of these reasons may be correct, but all overlook the obvious: the fact that he had sexual desires and fantasies, too. Freud showed little hesitancy in giving opinions about the psychodynamics of others, even those he never met, so he would have little grounds to object if we took the same liberties with him. After all, turnabout is fair play.

Remember, this was Vienna at about the turn of the century, a time of excessive modesty and guilt over taboo sexual thoughts. Just imagine Freud, a proper and healthy and sexually repressed young man himself, sequestered alone in an office with these defenseless and attractive young ladies for session after session, exploring their private, intimate thoughts and probably wrestling with his own fantasies, too. That a sexual genesis for their problems should suggest itself to him (or any robust male for that matter) in this setting isn't surprising, not just based on what the women revealed but on the intimacy of the therapeutic relationship. That Freud was capable of experiencing taboo feelings is evident from a letter he wrote to a close colleague in 1897, in which he reported having overly tender feelings toward his oldest daughter, Mathilde, in a dream, then citing this as evidence of the sexual proclivities of fathers toward daughters. But that he later should exonerate the accused fathers of sexually abusing their daughters (especially when he had claimed for years that he had evidence of their guilt) by attributing the presumed abuse to the imagination of the supposed victims, and then shift his attention to the equivalency of fantasy and fact, never to pursue his original observations again, likely meant that he was motivated by a powerful unconscious force that he neither wanted to acknowledge nor understand.

Though speculative, my notion of what likely happened to change Freud's mind is that in working with his neurotic young ladies, he himself struggled with the forbidden desire to seduce one or more of them. Under the circumstances, this would not be that unusual. After all, during the Middle Ages, exorcists knew about the great dangers of becoming possessed themselves after being closeted alone for long stretches of time with demoniacally possessed young ladies or nuns who, as a sign of their bewitchment, often acted seductively. Evidence that the Devil also had taken possession of the priests was naturally based on their later developing sexual feelings toward these women while trying to rid them of their demons.[8] If something of this nature happened with Freud, it could explain his strange conversion. That way, if the accounts of early seduction were based solely on the overactive imaginations of his clients—if these sexual fantasies were part of their psychopathology—then Freud needn't acknowledge his own unprofessional thoughts. He had established his own psychological alibi.

That Freud was not always totally in command of his own feelings seems clear by certain later behavior on his part. With an apparently clear conscience, he went on to do what he would not condone in others and what no competent psychotherapist nowadays would ever do, namely, undertake the extended psychoanalysis of his own daughter, Anna, who forewent marriage and followed in her father's footsteps by becoming a psychoanalyst herself, and eventually, the mother of child psychoanalysis. During her initial three-year course of psychoanalysis, and then, later, during another one-year span, she shared her most intimate dreams with him. The few dreams that we know about are revealing. Once she dreamt that she was defending a farm belonging to her and her father, but when she went to draw her saber against the enemy, she became ashamed that it was broken. On another occasion, she dreamt that the wife of a colleague rented an apartment across the street from her father in order to shoot him. On another occasion, she dreamed that her father was a king and she was a princess, and that people were trying to separate them by political intrigue. Of course, the interpretation of dreams is fraught with perils, especially since the interpretation may reveal more about the interpreter than the person dreaming. But these particular dreams invite speculation, mainly because they are as revealing, in their own way, as the dramatic symptoms of the bewitched family I described. Whatever rationalizations Freud gave for continuing in this unorthodox relationship, they could not have been his real reasons, whether known to him or not. As a result, many of the psychological truths Freud propounded were likely tainted by his own countertransference. I suspect that he could have benefitted from someone pointing out his therapeutic impropriety, but then who possibly was qualified to comment on the motivations of the founder of psychoanalysis? Besides, few people knew about this well-kept secret.

I asked Peter Gay, the author of the exhaustive biography of Sigmund Freud, what he knew about this relationship other than what he mentioned in his writings.[9] "What information is available on that? Did he keep notes? Did she keep notes?"

"If he kept notes, I didn't see them," he answered. "[And if she did,] I bet she destroyed them. I didn't see any."

"Wouldn't it have been his practice to keep notes on anybody he saw?" I say.

"Afterwards, sure."

"So it may well be that there are notes available but you didn't have access to them?" I found it intriguing that Freud, who kept such copious notes on all his patients, should leave no incriminating or exonerating information behind on this most remarkable relationship, the psychoanalysis of an unmarried daughter by her father.

"There are certain matters in his life that I left undecided," he responded.

Yet I couldn't let this unthinkable issue lie, as it apparently had over the years. I'm amazed that it hadn't been the subject of more scrutiny. If it was an entirely innocent and proper relationship, I shouldn't expect it to have been so secretive, never alluded to in public by either the father or the daughter and only rarely in private to a select few. The absence of documentation about what transpired can only fuel speculation. Also of great interest is what Freud's wife and his other children thought about this, but no one cared to ask. For someone who exposed so much of his fantasy life with others, he was remarkably mum about this psychoanalytic affair.

"Do you feel that Freud cultivated some kind of facade?" I asked Professor Gay at another point in our conversation.

"Sure," he answered, "although I would argue that a facade is a part of the self as well. . . . But from a psychoanalytic point of view, I certainly would like to think that you get beyond surface manifestations if you're lucky and persistent. Freud said, if you recall, in the Dora case, that nobody could keep a secret, and that a little truth will just ooze out from every pore of the person who is talking. You certainly can look for clues in silence. I tend to do that, as I think most historians in one way or the other do."

Yes, I thought, truth does ooze out, but not only from patients. Though highly unlikely that Freud's conscious intentions were anything less than caring and proper, his own silence about the analysis of his daughter blares out that something was going on inside him that wasn't strictly kosher.

PSYCHOLOGICAL TRUTHS

This leads us back to the nature and value of psychological truth. With so many people launched on a course of self-discovery, self-actualization, self-realization, and getting-in-touch-with-themselves, this issue holds special significance. A psychotherapeutic industry exists to meet these expectations, peopled with psychiatrists, counselors, psychotherapists of all persuasions, ministers, and guides, peddlers of assorted truths who offer their clientele the prospects of a better and less troubled life. Are these different and sometimes contradictory psychological truths really "true," and if not, does it matter?

One of the major problems with any insight-oriented psychotherapy based on the uncovering of important, early-life experiences is that it's difficult if not impossible to establish the historical truth through the customary exploration of your memories, fantasies, and dreams, no matter how thorough the probing or how long the treatment. This is so for a lot of reasons. For one, your memories and perceptions are designed to support your biases. You selectively remember or repress certain information, and many of your experiences are indescribable or difficult to translate into words. Your memories tend to be shaped by the theoretical outlook of your therapist. And you tend not to include disconfirming experiences in your accounts.

For these reasons, what you come to regard as historical truth really represents plausibility. This plausibility involves how well your account embraces all the pertinent elements of your experiences and how cohesive it seems.

What often adds conviction to your account is the element of drama, the experiencing of strong emotions during your recollections. The discharge of this pent-up emotionality—tears, joy, fear, anger—stamps your account with the imprimatur of authenticity and truth. That's why so many healing ceremonies, marathon therapy sessions, intensive insight-oriented techniques, and therapeutic encounters try to produce emotional arousal. When you're emotionally aroused, you're not only more suggestible but also more primed to accept what others say as gospel truth.

In his seminal work on the distinction between narrative and historical truth, Donald P. Spence examines the problems of establishing truth within the context of psychoanalytic investigations.[10] It is naive, he claims, to assume that the patient can be an unbiased reporter and the analyst an unbiased listener. Throughout psychotherapy, the patient deals with the conflict between what is true but hard to describe—that is, the pure memory—and what is describable but partly untrue—that is, the screen memory. The very attempt to translate the original memory destroys it because the words, as they are chosen, likely misrepresent the image, and because the translation, no matter how good, replaces the original. On the analyst's part, a complementary paradox takes place. The dilemma the analyst faces is how to get behind the patient's utterances to recover the original memory versus the easier solution of interpreting the utterances and leaving the memory behind. Resolution of this mutual paradox takes the form of a negotiated understanding between the patient and the analyst. The patient, like the poet or artist, must always be searching for the right expression, and the analyst, like the biographer, must always be trying to fathom the patient's intended meaning. This negotiated understanding represents narrative truth.

Explanatory systems or personal stories acquire narrative truth in several ways. The very process of putting confusing and ambiguous feelings into words gives the formulation a reality. Even in the absence of confirmatory memories, this formulation still offers a reason why certain events have happened. No matter how improbable the explanation, it tends to be treated as true if it provides missing links to account for otherwise complex and disjointed events. Pattern and coherence give the account credibility in its own right. By making what follows depend on what happened before, the narrative partly relieves patients from responsibility for their actions. Even when the reconstruction of the past is entirely imaginary, it acquires the mantle of truth if it lets patients find coherence and meaning in their personal stories and make sense out of their chaotic experiences. And it becomes officially true and sometimes more real than actual historical truth when an authoritative figure, such as their analyst, gives the narrative the stamp of approval.

In a sense, the task of psychotherapy is to offer you a more satisfactory life story or get you to move on in the one you already have. Mostly, you enter therapy when you're stuck in a certain chapter of your life and don't know what you want to do next or don't like what you see ahead for yourself. What a successful therapeutic experience does is to reestablish the narrative flow, reawaken a sense of meaning in your life, restore personal control, and realign you with the prevalent cultural myth. The very process of recounting a drama, in which you are the protagonist, to someone in a helping, parental role, such as a therapist, obliges you to push your personal narrative ahead.

With more doctrinaire therapeutic approaches, you don't have much personal narrating to do. Not only is the story explicitly spelled out for you but your role and script are as well. Alcoholics Anonymous, for example, promotes the sober life, tells you how to achieve and sustain it, and gives you slogans, formulas and behavioral proscriptions for preventing relapse. With less doctrinaire approaches, such as nondirective psychotherapy, most of the burden for constructing a suitable life story falls on you. You're granted more autonomy in deciding what course to pursue and choosing what roles to play. Common to all these approaches is the necessity for "reframing" or "recontextualizing" your life, placing it within a modified narrative structure that tells you what makes you tick and how best to get what you want. So depending on the therapeutic approach you adopt, your task is either to find a ready-made personal narrative that fits or to construct one of your own.

In short, a suitable therapeutic narrative represents story-telling at its best.[11] When gaps and discrepancies occur, when inconsistencies and contradictions exist, when the plot of your account seems too forced or shaky, the therapist has the task of helping you rewrite your personal narrative through interpretations, instructions, or reconstructions so that no disconfirming experiences exist.

That's why whatever benefit you receive from therapy doesn't depend on the particular theoretical orientation to which you're exposed, even though you tend to produce insights and confirmatory evidence to support it. Because your mental content is malleable and easily influenced by the explanatory system you adopt, your thoughts, dreams, and fantasies are likely to be colored by your therapist's orientation, either through your own desires to please your therapist or the therapist's need to indoctrinate you with his or her theoretical point of view. This likewise holds for any religious or political system or "ism" you're drawn to that lets you interpret your distress as a deviation from some ideal norm and that offers remedies to correct whatever is wrong.

For a variety of reasons, people have a need to shape their experiences to conform to the theoretical expectations of their therapists. This explains why the mental patients of Dr. J. M. Charcot, the famous nineteenth-century neurologist at the Salpetrière, reputedly hallucinated in several different languages, depending upon the nationalities of the renowned visitors who made rounds with him. This explains why patients undergoing psychoanalysis have Freudian dreams, those undergoing a Jungian analysis have mythic dreams pregnant with universal symbols and primitive archetypes, and those exposed to spiritual counseling have dreams with religious import. Sometimes patients unwittingly say things or have experiences simply to please the therapist, even when they don't necessarily believe what they report.

John Cheever, for example, was a master at performances of this sort. If his therapist wanted dreams, he gave him spicy dreams. If the therapist wanted family pathology, Cheever told lurid tales about what happened when he grew up. If the therapist wanted bedroom adventures, he told him the gory details of his many affairs. And according to Scott Donaldson, his biographer, if his therapist fancied schizophrenia, Cheever spoke of the two John Cheevers, the pretended and authentic one. But all the while he concealed certain truths from the psychiatrist and looked down on him for being taken in.

"What do you feel Cheever's gratification was with his boast about never telling his psychiatrist the truth," I asked Donaldson, who also wrote biographies about Ernest Hemingway and F. Scott Fitzgerald. "What was the game?"

"It fits in with what he was, which was an inventor of stories. It was probably not that much different for him to go to a psychiatrist than it would have been for him to go to lunch with a friend and see people across the room and start telling a story about them, although he'd never seen them before. It's just that with a psychiatrist, he's supposedly telling stories about himself and he's pretty much confined to those people who have most impinged on his life, but this is not going to keep him from inventing things. This is part of what makes these people more complicated than others. They are story-tellers, and we must expect them to tell stories about themselves just as they do about others.

"In Cheever's case, he's also trying to avoid any real confrontation with his behavior and problem, particularly his drinking. He really didn't want to face his demons directly at the time, and therefore he's doing what comes naturally to him, which is to provide entertainment."

What Scott Donaldson observed about his subject, Cheever himself confirmed in his *Journals*. "I have been a storyteller since the beginning of my life," he writes, "rearranging facts in order to make them more interesting and sometimes more significant. . . . I have improvised a background for myself—genteel, traditional—and it is generally accepted." [12]

John Cheever's imaginative productions in psychotherapy were far from unusual for a creative writer. There is something about the storytelling aspects of psychotherapy that encourage flights of fancy that often assume the mantle of truth—at least, until reality gets in the way. Somehow, in these situations, the truth becomes murky and reality becomes whatever the therapist and patient believe it to be. In a sense, this was the situation Freud faced when he was receptive to believing the accounts of early sexual abuse that his patients confirmed again and again. When he closed his mind to this reality, he then began to find that their confessions of abuse simply reflected their unconscious forbidden wishes.

During Anne Sexton's psychotherapy, we find a crystallization of this very dilemma, and one that Freud's apologists may cite as justification for his abandoning his seduction theory. In writing her biography of Anne Sexton, Diane Middlebrook had access to the therapist's tapes and notes of her subject during her therapy sessions.[13] These sources of information are invaluable for the light they cast on the nature of psychotherapeutic truth.

Early in Anne Sexton's therapy, a new persona, Elizabeth, heralded her appearance, while Sexton was in a hypnotic trance, by scrawling messages in the handwriting of a child. This entity then began to appear more frequently, sometimes ludicrously typing letters in the dark so that Anne, her bodily host, could not see them. It was through Elizabeth that Sexton's psychiatrist first learned that she had been sexually abused by her father as a child.

Although Sexton's psychiatrist made a point of identifying Elizabeth as a persona and not an alter personality, I have reservations about this fine distinction. So I asked Diane Middlebrook, Sexton's biographer, about this. "As you came to know her through the materials and so on, did you see her as having multiple selves or did you see her as more coherent?"

"That episode of her playing with an identity, called Elizabeth, was obviously entertaining as well as frightening to her. She came to draw upon that ability to be a lot of people, as a performer does and as an actress does, so what was initially a disorienting experience was transformed into a gift."

Although her propensity to dissociate and to sexualize relationships was typical for a sexually abused woman, it was not so easy for her therapist to establish whether the abuse actually happened. Her recollections about being molested came at a time when she was writing a play about incest and, as she herself would comment, once she put a scene into words, the words often became the reality. "I wouldn't make this all up, or I don't exist at all." And during a later therapy session, she asked, "Or do I make up a trauma to go with my symptoms?"[14] probably unaware that her question was central to the same issues Freud struggled with.

For a time, her therapist dealt with this supposed incest as a real event because it was real for her, a metaphor for various personal conflicts, even though he did not believe the event really happened. He said that he let this new persona, Elizabeth, communicate to help Sexton deal with the feelings she wanted to split off. But in time, when he became concerned that his patient was dangerously close to developing a full-blown multiple personality, he dropped his interest in Elizabeth. Soon afterward, Elizabeth disappeared and never emerged again.

Later, Sexton herself would identify this episode with Elizabeth as a "truth crime," an invention to express a repressed part of herself. She also admitted faking total amnesia of this persona to her psychiatrist. She said she had "no self" so she produced a different one for different people. "I would rather have a double personality than be a total lie," she revealed.[15] She also confessed to being "nothing, if not an actress off the stage, . . . that there is no true part of me. . . . I will permit my therapy and think it all interesting as long as it doesn't touch me. I am a story-maker. . . ."[16]

Interestingly, her powers of invention, which may have hampered her therapy, were marvelously suited for her art. In her trances, she sometimes was a channel for lies, but at her typewriter, she was a channel for poetry. The symptoms of her mental illness, according to her biographer, were like metaphors, containing meanings laden with personal history. Anne Sexton herself later likened her creative mind to an analyst who "gives pattern and meaning to what the person sees as only incoherent experience."[17]

There are several observations we should make about this particular episode in Sexton's therapy, some of which seem paradoxical. Her therapist kept allowing Elizabeth to emerge in trance even though he believed her to be a fabrication and let her talk about being abused by her father as a child even though he doubted that this happened. Anne Sexton continued to flirt with her new persona, even claiming amnesia for her appearance, even though she knew that these experiences weren't real and that she was manufacturing memories and imbuing them with truth. Both the therapist and patient seemed engaged in a peculiar transaction, a *folie a deux* of sorts, communicating about events that neither believed to be so.

What the therapist and patient both seemed to be doing was constructing a suitable narrative structure in which both could comfortably participate. The therapist put his patient into a trance, which presumably was under his control, but this seemingly dependent patient, by her dramatic productions, continued to lead her therapist along. Both parties apparently felt comfortable engaging in this mutual fiction until the new personality threatened to become real.

In a sense, the process of psychotherapy is an attempt on both the part of the therapist and the patient to impose order on chaos. It's easy for people to become disoriented with their inner fantasy world in which images rapidly transform, where time is meaningless, and where the landscapes are colored and shaped by personal needs. Most therapeutic explanatory systems serve as road maps, identifying the meaning of symbols and explaining where patients have been and are heading, and offer rituals for coping with unpleasant feelings during the trip. Without suitable road maps, it's easy for people to get lost.

What this therapy vignette about Anne Sexton also points out is the sometimes reciprocal relationship between the psychotherapeutic process and creativity. In therapy, her acts of invention led her therapist and her in circles; in her personal storytelling, they produced noteworthy poetry. In therapy, the therapist was the final judge of her productions; in her poetry, her own judgment was what counted. In therapy, the contents of her communications were bound by the constraints of the theoretical system and confined to the therapy hour; in her creative activity, she could select the rules and write what she pleased. In therapy, all therapeutic insights, so to speak, led back to Rome. Most of the answers were known beforehand. In contrast, the creative process sought new explanations or presentations, mostly of a highly personal nature, for existing facts.

Aside from representing a metaphor for certain unexpressed feelings, the emergence of a new persona in Anne Sexton's therapy also represented a failure of the psychotherapeutic process to address what was bothering her at the time. If she had been able to communicate her chaotic feelings adequately, Sexton wouldn't have needed to create an alter self. What this suggests is that the psychotherapeutic system was lacking. If it was adequate, it should have reined in all her loose emotional fragments and incorporated them within the therapeutic narrative without her having a part of her split off.

HALLMARKS OF A THERAPEUTIC NARRATIVE

What, then, are the distinguishing features of a therapeutic narrative—or any ideology or belief system, for that matter—that lets you understand your problems and gives you a sense of control over them? For a therapeutic narrative to be beneficial, it must be characterized by continuity, consistency, conformity, and confirmation, which, incidentally, also represent the hallmarks for all sound biographies and literary narratives. In the absence of any or all of these features, your insights aren't likely to endure.[18]

CONTINUITY

"Continuity" means that the personal narrative adopted by you needs to be continuous within the context of your culture and times. Demoniacal explanations for psychological disturbances, for example, which were fashionable in the Middle Ages, are no longer so, except in certain subcultures. Likewise, what may be true for you as a Westerner may not be true for you if you were born in Asia or Saudi Arabia. Personal narratives that lack continuity lack durability—not only because of the emotional disruptiveness of discontinuities but also because continuities have a momentum of their own. This is why people usually prefer to cling to the continuity of their present life, no matter how miserable it seems, rather than risk the uncertainty that major change may bring.

Continuity also lets your life story move forward in time, with the past preceding the present and the present preceding the future. It's possible, perhaps even likely, that time as you know it doesn't exist, and that your personal history represents an artifact of your biological development. Since you progress sequentially from birth, to childhood, to adulthood, to old age, to death, you're biologically programmed to interpret what transpires during your lifetime along this temporal dimension. Continuity lets you believe that you're the same person from inception to death, that all your experiences belong to you, and that no real discontinuities exist in your life, despite sleep, amnesias, or unconsciousness.

Because continuity represents a progression over time, it artificially generates a sense of personal growth during psychotherapy. Surely, all that you experienced, all that you brought to light, all that you've come to understand about yourself has contributed to your growing maturity. Or so you're inclined to tell yourself. The question, perhaps unanswerable, is whether this perception of yourself is illusory or real.

Let me highlight this issue. After many years of soul-searching, I see myself as a drastically different person now than before. Yet when an old friend visits, he says after we spend fifteen minutes together, "It's really incredible—you haven't changed a bit." Shaken, I wonder whether it's possible after all these years, after so many learning experiences, important encounters with others, therapeutic interactions of various sorts, job changes, major shifts in political beliefs and a growing maturity and wisdom that I can be basically the same. I also feel more at peace with myself. Besides, I don't want to be the immature person I was years ago, filled with doubts and insecurities. Surely, those who see me the same can't be very perceptive, since I know I've changed in so many basic ways. But then I wonder. Is my perception of personal growth also a myth, a convenient fiction that lets me believe I have more control over fashioning myself than I do, or did I really change in any fundamental sense? Or am I simply the same person I've always been but only further along in my personal life story than before?

This sense of continuity affects you in other ways as well. Because your life moves forward in time, you're more disposed to rue the loss of your future with your death than to grieve over those who died before your birth. It makes as much logical sense for you to be saddened that you didn't know the many generations of your progenitors whose traits and dispositions you express as to be saddened by your ignorance of the future generations who will bear your genes. Though you may show interest in your family roots, you do so more to establish a connectedness than to grieve over a loss. The future belongs to you, the past to your ancestors. Yet your parents and grandparents and great-grandparents are just as much a part of you as your children, grandchildren, and great-grandchildren. And your nonexistence before your conception is just as much of a nonexistence as your nonexistence after your death. Therefore, it makes as much sense to believe you existed in the distant past as to believe you will continue to exist in the far future.

Even the comforting belief in reincarnation, while accommodating both the past and future, doesn't eliminate the sadness over future loss. Buddhist lore holds that you must drink from the soup bowl of forgetfulness before each reincarnation, with complete loss of all memory for your previous life. The promise of reincarnation is attractive but presents certain paradoxes about who you think you are. If you inhabit a different body and possess a different brain and have no recollection of experiences of a past life, are you the same or different person with each rebirth? If you're different, then reincarnation offers little solace for the perpetuation of your self. If you're the same person, then all the personal experiences and memories you've gathered over a lifetime make no difference for who you are. Or, stretching possibilities, if you're simultaneously both the same and different person, then the person you think you are both is and isn't you.

CONSISTENCY

A suitable therapeutic narrative also should be consistent. "Consistency" means that your story line needs to be coherent, comprehensive, and organized, that the plot hangs together, and that the disparate elements in your life are convincingly incorporated and accounted for in the narrative. The best explanatory systems therefore are those based on premises that, once accepted, lead to certain inevitable conclusions or which, much in the nature of the Hegelian dialectic, accommodate all contradictions. In psychoanalysis, for example, basic concepts such as symbolization, reaction formation, and the equivalence of opposites in the unconscious allow almost anything to mean anything you want within the context of your narrative structure. If you're receptive to the therapist's interpretation, then you're insightful; if not, then you are resistive and show denial. This is so for most comprehensive explanatory systems of human nature. As long as you can reason deductively, from accepted premises to conclusions you want to adopt, with defective logic or not, then you can make your personal narrative a self-confirming system, continually convincing yourself of its utility and truth. Thinking is a lot easier if you know your conclusions beforehand and where all reasoning must lead.

CONFORMITY

Then there is "conformity," which means that for your insights and explanations to gain authoritative import, they need to agree with the essential orientation of your therapist, counselor, shaman, religious leader, political ideologue, healer, or in a broader sense, societal or cultural myths. Enormous personal and social pressures are at work to mold your observations and experiences into a language acceptable to the outside authority—to tell that authority what he or she wants to hear so that the authority can look after your needs and then tell you what you want to hear. Past studies show that therapists, often unwittingly, exert a powerful influence over the verbal productions of their patients with such nonverbal cues as uh-huhs, grunts, nods, raised eyebrows, glances at the clock, as well as actual comments. With these reinforcers, they train you to produce personal stories that conform to their preconceived theoretical notions of psychological causality and that, in the process, confirm their beliefs. So you find yourself telling a story that binds the attention of your therapist, or if that doesn't suit you, find another therapist whose explanatory system is more compatible with what you are inclined to hear. In effect, then, an unknowing conspiracy of sorts develops in which you and your therapist work at constructing a narrative that suits both of your needs.

CONFIRMATION

The last criterion of a sound therapeutic narrative is "confirmation." Confirmation means that whatever insights you glean from therapy require approval by family, friends, colleagues or society, as well as continuing validation by yourself. Because of your tendency to revert to old ways of thinking over time or under duress, you have to keep seeking confirmation for your newfound beliefs. One common way you confirm your beliefs is by interpreting every success as a sign that your understanding is true and every failure as evidence that you aren't applying what you know, or there is more for you to learn.

THE MISSING INGREDIENTS

It would be misleading to give the impression that any therapeutic narrative that meets all these criteria will automatically relieve personal distress and bring contentment. In many instances, psychotherapies fail, even for those who are highly motivated and have recourse to the most experienced therapists. Anne Sexton, Ernest Hemingway, and Sylvia Plath, for instance, committed suicide despite many years of therapy and the availability of creative outlets. The issue is, what went wrong or what was overlooked?

Of course, it isn't possible to know all the factors contributing to such dire acts or even a poor therapeutic response, but we can make some educated guesses. The first is to state the obvious. The retrospective nature of most insight-oriented therapies makes them more suitable for reconstructing the past than for shaping the future. Therapists and patients alike operate under the same constraints as biographers who can't write the next chapter of their subjects' lives until they are in full possession of the facts and know what happens. Whatever control you have over certain aspects of the future may be largely on a *post hoc* or *ad hoc* basis, which aligns what transpired with what your expectations happen to be.

Another reason that therapeutic narratives fail is that some are appropriate under certain situations and not others. The momentous insights, for example, of the alcoholics and drug addicts whom I treated with LSD were impressive in a hospital setting, but had little relevance to the kinds of problems and difficulties they would encounter once they were back on the streets and caught up in their former lives. Being reborn, whether by drugs or spiritual healing, is no assurance that someone is better equipped to face life.

An older followup study of people who were reborn, healed or saved during religious conversions showed that about 90 percent backslid within two weeks.[19] This didn't deter them from experiencing another rebirth in the future. While the relapse rates for most forms of insight-oriented psychotherapy are probably far less, they are likely due to similar causes. The most likely reason for relapse is that the therapeutic narrative is not compelling, convincing, cogent, or comprehensive enough to explain away their problems, or override certain ingrained, habitual ways of responding. This reflects both on the adequacy of the particular psychotherapeutic system and the particular nature of the problems. No matter what people tell themselves or believe, certain problems may be resistant to the healing benefits of insights. They simply may not be able to talk themselves out of a deep depression or a severe panic attack or a habitual, morbid outlook, even when they think they know the reasons. A child who sees both of his parents murdered, a drunken teenager who accidentally kills someone in a car wreck, a woman who endures terrible privations and abuse in a concentration camp, or a young man exposed to the horrors of war may not be able to put aside these awful experiences completely, no matter the adequacy of the treatment narrative. The conventional narrative of learning-to-lead-an-ordinary-life may not be able to satisfactorily incorporate such extraordinary discontinuities within it, which, by their very nature, impede any ordinary, narrative flow. In these instances, the therapeutic task is to help these individuals find meaning in their stupefying experiences so that they can get on with the process of living.

Another way to put this is that the stories people have lived are sometimes too powerful to be modified substantially by reframing their experiences so that they seem more favorable or by any of the usual therapeutic narratives that their therapists or they embrace. Early psychological trauma, chemical imbalances within their brains, their basic temperaments, or their genetic makeups also may make them resistant to the potential benefits of most therapeutic narratives alone. In Hemingway's case, for instance, with a father who shot himself and a grandfather who almost did, or in Anne Sexton's case, with mentally ill relatives, two of whom committed suicide, the compelling nature of the family drama, like the inevitability of a Greek tragedy, may impel the protagonists to pursue their own self-destruction, even while they know they are doing it and maybe even know the reason why.

Perhaps the biggest failing of psychotherapy is that it can't give you what you want most, even though you try to avoid thinking about this. Aside from all your personal conflicts, unrealistic ambitions, and self-doubts, you're confronted with the potential meaninglessness of your existence and the finiteness of your self. In some fashion, this touches directly or indirectly on almost every problem you face. Most insight-oriented psychotherapies and self-help approaches recoil from issues of this sort, since they threaten their fundamental assumptions, all of which are designed to inculcate you with certain cultural myths about the nature of the self that allow you to reintegrate yourself into society. If all seems meaningless, you're asked to generate your own meaning by committing yourself to worthwhile projects and finding more appealing things to do. If you feel personally insignificant, you're assured that you're precious and important. If you become emotionally paralyzed by the eventuality of your death, you're told that you shouldn't worry about something you have no control over but instead should make the most out of the time you have left. And if you're struck by the absurdity of it all—the wars, human cruelty, disease, starvation, suffering and pain, and senseless struggles for power—you're encouraged to try to make the world a better place to live in, or to look at the positive side of things. These are all reasonable messages, and ones you're usually primed to hear. But sometimes they aren't convincing.

These shortcomings of psychotherapy shouldn't be taken as an indictment of it. After all, it has an impossible task. It has to shift your concerns from inevitabilities you can do nothing about and mysteries you can't fathom to the artificialities of social life and the mundane practicalities of living. With these constraints, it's remarkable that it's as effective as it is. Even when you continue doing much of what you always did, feeling much of what you always felt, thinking much of what you always thought, the very act of corraling your experiences and doubts within a therapeutic narrative is often sufficient to let you feel more control over where your personal story will lead.

EIGHT

How Did
Hitler Live
With Himself?

Ｈｏｗ ｄｏ ｗｅ ｉｎｃｏｒｐｏｒａｔｅ ｅｖｉｌ into our conception of the self? Is "original sin" inherent in human nature, or do we come into this world innocent and pure, corrupted only by bad child-rearing or social inequities? Whether we believe that we've been born with evil or have acquired it, we typically resist accepting it as part of us. Evil represents corruption, defect, and degradation, and challenges any idealized notion of the self. To rid ourselves of this imperfection, we engage in various purifying acts, such as confession, atonement, or punishment. If we can't accept responsibility for our wickedness, we attribute it to some external agency, like the Devil, or conveniently wall it off from memory. If that option isn't suitable, we find justification for our immorality, or recast it as good. Or, in the postmodernist spirit, we may even try to eliminate the very existence of personal evil by viewing it as a metaphor for the various political, social, or psychological forces impinging on us.[1]

These typical ways of dealing with personal evil suggest that we've arrived at an uneasy accommodation with it. If not inherent to human nature, evil is at least common to it. Pride, avarice, lust, envy, gluttony, anger, and sloth, otherwise known as the seven deadly sins, underlie a host of social transgressions, but they are failings that we accept as distinctly human. Admonitions, such as "He that is without sin among you, let him first cast a stone," or "There but for the grace of God go I," remind us of our close kinship with sinners and a need for charity toward them.

But this notion of evil as a common moral shortcoming overlooks an important distinction. However apt, it fails to penetrate into the very heart of darkness and differentiate between evil and EVIL. It doesn't deal with horrific acts that are beyond comprehension and that strike us as inhuman: not just "ordinary" murder but massacres and atrocities, not only cruelty toward others but torturing and mutilating them, not only violating others' human rights but treating them as subhuman. It offers no understanding of crimes that even a merciful God couldn't forgive, and if He did, could weaken our belief in Him. Most important, even though we may be willing to acknowledge the "human-ness" of moral imperfection, it doesn't reveal whether people capable of such abominations have anything in common with us, and if they do, what that says about us.

As our initial focus of attention we can turn to two people who represent the personification of evil for many. Adolf Hitler was responsible for killing about six million Jews and several million other "misfits," and for launching a war that claimed over twelve million more civilian lives. Joseph Stalin, especially through his repression of White Russians and kulaks (merchants and other enterprising persons), initiated a policy that was responsible for an estimated forty million civilian deaths.[2] Add to that the systematic oppression and torture and cruelty inflicted on many millions more, and we have crimes against humanity that boggle the imagination.

With evil of this magnitude, our challenge is to find out how people like Hitler and Stalin managed to live with themselves. Unfortunately, this is partic-ularly difficult to do since these were two of the most secretive men in history. Hitler claimed more than once, "You will never know what I am thinking." Within his inner circle, Albert Speer, his chief architect and later Minister of Armaments, was his only confidante, and a limited one at that. "If Hitler had been capable of friendship," Speer told Alan Bullock, who interviewed him at length after he came out of prison, "I think I would have been his best friend, his only friend." As for Stalin, who literally rewrote Russian history, page by page, he let only his daughter, Svetlana, get close to him, until they eventually became estranged. Others risked death if they had too much personal knowl-edge.

Because of the limited personal information available on these leaders, I asked Alan Bullock, author of the authoritative biography *Hitler and*

Stalin: Parallel Lives, what questions he would ask the two men that might help to understand them better, if he had an opportunity to interview them during an unguarded moment.

"We're dealing with people outside the range of normal experience," he replied, in response to this hypothetical scenario. "They're still human beings. I'm not getting away from that. But they never would have agreed to an interview unless they could dominate it for their own purpose. They simply wouldn't have talked. You'd never have gotten in.

"All you could have done would be to take Hitler through his well-known act. He held a very coherent view about human history based on his racist beliefs. Once you start on that line, and accept his assumptions about inferior and superior races, it's a logical view.

"Stalin had an equally fixed view. . . . He used the Marxist clichés about class warfare, the things that Lenin had said before about Revolutions . . . many people will die, millions of people."

I asked Charles Bracelen Flood, who documented Hitler's rise in his book, *Hitler: The Path to Power*, to conduct the same hypothetical interview with his subject, Adolf Hitler.[3] "I don't think (Hitler) could give me the answer to the most important question any more than Beethoven could in a different way," he responded. "Hitler was a genius. He was an evil genius, but that does not take away the fact that he was a genius. I don't believe geniuses can tell you where it comes from, how it operates. He once was quoted as saying that he moved like a sleep-walker. What he meant was that sometimes he didn't know why he did things, or why he did them when he did them, or just how he did them. But again and again they were extraordinarily successful.

"Here you have arguably the most obscure man in Germany, not even a German citizen, an Austrian, coming into the arena—believe me, there were plenty of contenders for political power on the right and the left at the close of World War I—and having this remarkable rise to power. I think there is more here than just attributes, such as intelligence or some shrewdness or this or that. There is something there that you would be very foolish to say 'Now we've got it fully analyzed and quantified.'"

So now we face our first dilemma. We hope to understand the motivations and mental processes of people who not only are secretive but who fabricate information about themselves. It's difficult enough to figure out why people like Anne Sexton lied, or Katherine Anne Porter invented her past, or John Cheever made the therapeutic process a game, but now we have people who simply don't want others to know who they were before they came to power, and were willing to kill others to make sure they didn't find out. To complicate matters, we also have to deal with the unfathomable aspects of genius. These are formidable obstacles. Still, there are many things we can glean.

WERE HITLER AND STALIN "HUMAN"?

Before we can know how people like Hitler and Stalin managed to live with themselves, we have to establish that they were not freaks of Nature, humans but somehow not "human." When we examine the lives of these individuals before they rose to absolute power, we find little to suggest they were aberrations of the human species or that clearly forecasted the evil they later would perpetrate. In fact, before their ascent to power, most people who knew them saw them as quite ordinary and didn't take them seriously. Probably the traits that separated them from most others—their unbounded ambition and supreme confidence in themselves—were not so obvious to others at the time, or if they were, didn't strike them as pathological.

BEGINNINGS

Though Hitler and Stalin generally denied others access to information about their pasts, we do know some things about them. We can speculate, as others have done, that Stalin's mistrust of other people partly stemmed from the many physical beatings he received during his childhood from a father who drank heavily and also beat his wife, and that his feeling of specialness came from his mother who invested all her hopes and ambitions in him. Because of her aspirations for him, he was sent to the church school and then to the theological college to become a priest rather than sent off to learn a cobbler's trade, as his father proposed. Becoming increasingly attracted to the Marxist notion of a class war that would overthrow the corrupt social order, he quit the seminary at the age of twenty to devote himself to politics after being branded as a troublemaker. Marxism seemed a perfect fit for his psychological and intellectual needs—it offered a supposed scientific basis for the realization of a utopian society, and it replaced the dogmatic theology he couldn't accept with a new orthodoxy and intolerance for dissent. It was during these early years that he fashioned his new identity, assuming the name of a Caucasian outlaw/hero, Koba, and later identifying with Lenin, a revolutionary hero, by adopting the name of Stalin, which meant "man of steel."

During his childhood, Adolf Hitler did not have to endure the hardships and poverty that Stalin did. His father was a relatively successful, thrice-married civil servant who left his family reasonably well provided for after he died. Like Stalin, Hitler was a choirboy, but in a Benedictine monastery. His father, though authoritarian by certain accounts, wasn't physically abusive (although Hitler claimed his father often whipped him), and his mother, from all accounts, was affectionate toward him. In school, though reasonably bright, he resisted the discipline of regular studies and only showed a special interest in art. In his late teens, he began to view himself as a heroic rebel. His own hero was Richard Wagner, whom he claimed to be his only forerunner. Unfortunately for the world, his image of himself as an artistic genius was thwarted when he failed his entrance examination at the Vienna Academy of Arts, and the director suggested that his talents lay in architecture and not in painting. Uncertain about his future, especially after another failed attempt to enter the Academy, he joined the army and fought in the war—a time he called the happiest of his life—and then experienced the bitterness of Germany's defeat. After he left the Army, he was drawn to politics, perhaps because he had no other occupational prospects at the time, and dedicated himself to bringing glory back to his country and revenging its defeat. Wandering about and observing the social tensions in pre-World War II Vienna, Hitler later claimed in *Mein Kampf*, he began to shape his world view. He knew what had to be done. His epiphany was that Marxism and Jewry represented the threats to his beloved Germany.

FRIENDSHIP AND INTIMACY

What do we know about Hitler's and Stalin's ability to form close relations with others? Although both showed the capacity for affection, its display was rare and its effects often were destructive. When he was sixteen, Hitler became intimate friends with August Kubizek, who was studying piano at the time. Though he claimed not to have loved his father, Hitler seemed deeply and sincerely devoted to his mother and terribly distressed when she died after a painful and lingering bout with cancer. At age seventeen, he wrote love poems to a young woman named Stephanie, who never responded, and made declarations of suicide when she became engaged to someone else. He was infatuated with Geli Raubal, his niece, who was twenty years his junior, and became jealous of her. When she committed suicide, supposedly to escape his possessiveness (although certain accounts say he shot her in a fit of rage), he became disconsolate and refused to drink alcohol or eat meat for the remainder of his life. Before his rise to power, he formed a close friendship with Ernst Röhm, whom he later had put to death. As dictator, he formed a liaison with Eva Braun, but her diary complained of his neglect and humiliating treatment of her. During the course of their relationship, she made two suicide attempts, and when he took his life, she also took her own.

Those closest to Stalin also seemed destined for suicide and misery. After his second wife committed suicide, he refused to go to her funeral or visit her grave and claimed that she left him as an enemy. His youngest son died an alcoholic at forty-one. When Yakov, Stalin's older son, learned that his father branded him a traitor because he surrendered to the Germans in the early part of the war, he committed suicide by running against an electric fence in a prison camp. The only person Stalin let himself be close to was his daughter, Svetlana, but they eventually became estranged when she grew older and tried to lead her own life.

So were Hitler and Stalin capable of caring for others? The answer is a qualified "Yes." Hitler sometimes seemed touched by certain kinds of suffering and could show consideration for his staff. He fed birds and tried to reduce the pain of lobsters being boiled alive. Though he could order the extermination of the feeble-minded without compunction, he remembered his secretaries' birthdays and was generous toward those who helped him when he was poor. *"When I think about it,"* he amazingly claimed, *"I realize that I'm extraordinarily humane."*[4] Stalin could care for his first wife and his daughter, and Hitler could care for his niece and mistress, but only to the extent that these women let themselves be completely dominated by them. Hitler seemed genuinely distraught by his mother's death, but Stalin, who seemed to have a good relationship with his mother, didn't attend her funeral. Whatever their feelings toward the women in their lives, both men held women in little regard as individuals and had strong views about their fulfilling traditional female roles.

Whereas they seemed to regard women as possessions, they mostly viewed other men as threats. Hitler inspired intense loyalty among those in his inner circle, while Stalin produced allegiance based on fear. Hitler seemed fond of Albert Speer, with whom he shared his grand visions, and trusted a few others, such as Himmler and Göring, while Stalin remained suspicious of everyone. Neither, though, seemed genuinely interested in establishing intimate relationships with others based on any semblance of equality. In the discourse between them, there was little give and take. Hitler pontificated, and the others listened; unless he had a particular interest in what they had to say, he didn't want to hear their points of view. Up until he wielded absolute power, Stalin was calculating about everything he said and deeply suspicious about the motives of others. Neither he nor Hitler tolerated opposition or dissent about matters that mattered to them. Their main interest in others was in whether they represented potential dangers or whether they could facilitate their plans.

"Do you have any sense about what Hitler and Stalin might have been hiding, why they were so secretive, what was that terrible, personal information that they were guarding at all cost?" I asked Alan Bullock.

"They did not believe in trust. Hitler probably was more trusting of relationships. He was a much more secure personality than Stalin. And he knew that he had this charismatic power. I don't think Stalin had that at all. He ruled by fear, not by charisma. He was distrustful, to the point where he regarded every man as his enemy, and looked with paranoid eyes to see them everywhere. He actually wiped out nearly all his contemporaries in the Bolshevik party.

"Now Hitler was different from that. He would never trust any man with his own thoughts. But on the other hand, he was not insecure. Göring and Himmler were in fact faithful to the very end. Hitler trusted them. He didn't tell them anything. He kept his secrets to himself. To some degree, on the other hand, he was perfectly frank about seeking to gain power and using it to restore Germany to the leading position in Europe. Both men (Hitler and Stalin) gained enormously from the fact that people didn't take them seriously until it was too late."

"Do you think that from your study of Hitler that there was anyone who *really* knew him?" I asked Charles Bracelen Flood.

"I would say no," he answered, "one reason being that I don't think he knew himself very well, and that was what the love of violence was all about. He probably was incapable of showing very much of himself to anyone."

"How might he describe himself?" I asked, hypothetically.

"He would have this myth of himself . . . that he, the humble soldier, fought on the Western front and felt called to do this for Germany. And then he would launch into an historically false although widely believed idea that it was a Jewish-Marxist conspiracy that had stabbed Germany in the back at the end of the war. He would tell you that having fought on the battlefield, he felt more the need to fight the traitors that were stabbing the brave soldiers and the good German rank and file at home in the back. He'd really get sort of a Joan of Arc thing. He would say his mission was to save the German people in their hour of crisis and humiliation and need and poverty and so forth after the war. He would then expand about all he did to save and help Germany, and with it would come a very callous disregard for the lives of those very same Germans.

"There was a point in the second World War where somebody said to him, in effect, 'Führer, I'm sure you feel so badly about the thousands who are dying at Stalingrad, the thousands of young soldiers.' Hitler just looked blank and said, 'Well, that's what young soldiers are for,' meaning, to be killed or sacrificed. So we may have a man with a sense of history, in which he sees himself so firmly placed that a hundred thousand lives here or there are really of no consequence. The big thing is Germany, its destiny, and how he is bringing that destiny about."

HISTORIC ROLE

If anything was distinctive about these people, it was their almost messianic sense of mission. But grandiosity of this sort is hardly indicative of evil. It often is found in people who aspire to great deeds: religious prophets, composers, scientists, creative artists, and the like. It also is not uncommon in leaders of democratic nations. Charles de Gaulle, for example, claimed that he *was* France ("*Je suis la France*") and that he was destined to save the French nation during and after World War II. Later, after liberating Paris, he proclaimed, "I felt I was fulfilling a function beyond myself. . . . I was an instrument of destiny." In his assessment of de Gaulle, Jean-Paul Sartre wryly observed, "I do not believe in God. But if I had to choose between God and de Gaulle, I would vote for God. He is more modest."

As did de Gaulle, both Hitler and Stalin saw themselves as agents of destiny. Hitler believed in his own infallibility. He claimed that he was chosen by Providence to restore the German people to their rightful place as the master race after their humiliating defeat in World War I. He aspired to create mankind anew. Stalin sought to end Russia's backwardness by making it the first socialist state in the world. He saw himself as the sole interpreter of Marxist-Leninist doctrine. To achieve these historic goals, human sacrifice was necessary. History would forgive the suffering and deaths of untold millions because, in the end, the common people—the *volk* for Hitler, or the *proletariat* for Stalin—would benefit, and the entire world would be a better place.

Both Hitler and Stalin had a need to dominate, and each manipulated the public in his own way. Hitler, through his personal charisma, could shape the expectations of the public, and because of his ability to read its mood, receive affirmation of the myth he created. Originally, Stalin gained power through his identification with Lenin, a type of apostolic succession, but in time, he was content to rule through terror and fear. As consummate politicians, both Hitler and Stalin, taking advantage of modern technology, were able to transmit their created public images everywhere and thereby mold public opinion. Obedience was not enough for Stalin; he wanted to control everyone's thoughts. The Hitler myth and the Stalin cult transformed each of them into messiahs who could offer eventual salvation for their people.

As these leaders gained absolute power, they assumed god-like status. With no checks to their omnipotent fantasies, they could impose their world view on the populace and eliminate anybody who stood in their way. Under these conditions, conscience became a handicap, "a Jewish invention, a blemish like circumcision," according to Hitler. Ruthlessness became a virtue, since it led to a quicker implementation of goals, and suspiciousness toward others was adaptive since enemies with agendas of their own lurked everywhere. "Providence has ordained that I should be the greatest liberator of humanity," Hitler claimed. "I am freeing man from . . . the dirty and degrading self-mortification of a chimera called conscience and morality."[5]

For both Hitler and Stalin, the blending of their personal selves and world views offered personal life stories with acceptable rationales for everything they did. Personal guilt was irrelevant if one acted on behalf of a noble cause. Capitalizing partly on the alien appearance and differentness of members of fundamentalist Jewish sects, Hitler not only cast Jews as a separate race but blamed them for Germany's humiliating defeat in the war and for the perceived decadence in society. Rid society of the Jew, he claimed, and the Teutonic race would be purified. Whether his view was born of a personal, virulent anti-Semitism or was calculated is difficult to say, since he explicitly wrote in *Mein Kampf* that the art of leadership was to focus the attention of people on a single adversary. In any event, it was a shrewd political move. Stalin, in contrast, saw his greatest threat in the bourgeoisie and the kulaks, but he considered any individuals or groups, including his close associates, as enemies if he thought they stood in the way of his attempt to transform Russia into a utopian, socialist society.

"Are you saying you feel that their set of values is a determining feature that distinguishes Hitler and Stalin from other human beings?" I asked Alan Bullock.

"Yes. But I don't think it distinguishes enough. The Nazis had a mass following, so I don't think we can just say Hitler is unique. He was unique in his charismatic power and the power to move audiences, and he was exceptional in the power of will he showed. For example, from the time of Stalingrad, from January 1943 until May 1945, he forced the war to continue. He rejected any suggestion that promised peace. Again and again, he said, 'My luck will change.' Millions died. The German army was called upon to display remarkable discipline and suffer great losses as it retreated two thousand kilometers from Stalingrad to Berlin and did not break, which is a fantastic thing. It was the will of one man that held that in place.

"Stalin is a very different picture. He was much less secure than Hitler. Hitler was suspicious on general principles. He thought you should never tell anybody anything more than they needed to know to carry out orders, but he wasn't suspicious from a sense of personal insecurity. Take the period in the later 1920s, when he is no more than a marginal figure in German politics. Yet he's absolutely convinced that he will dominate Germany, and the people around him believe him. From the time he comes out of prison at the end of 1925 until the elections of September 1930, there was absolutely nothing really to encourage him. So he has a great strength in himself, and to the very end he says, 'Providence will intervene to save me.' Pale and shaken, the first thing he said to Mussolini on July 20th, 1944, after the failed assassination attempt, when the bomb exploded and Hitler was knocked about and bruised, was, 'Duce, this is proof that I am under the protection of Providence.' He believed it.

"Stalin was openly scornful of anything like a God or Providence. In his case the place of Providence was taken by the Marxist historical process. He identified himself with that. Both men claimed they were geniuses. The point is, Hitler said, 'I'm a genius,' and that was it; but Stalin said 'I'm a genius,' then he looked around to see if they all agreed, and if he saw the tremor of an eyelid, that man was marked."

"Other than labeling themselves geniuses, what other labels do you think they might have applied to themselves?"

"They thought they were men of destiny. Hitler clearly speaks of himself in the same terms as Napoleon and Bismarck and the great historical figures. Stalin sees himself as the heir of Lenin, but he also sees himself as the heir of Czar Peter the Great, Czar Ivan the Terrible, both of whom fascinated him. Stalin is different from Hitler in another respect. Hitler can be quite open about what he believes. He speaks and acts in accordance with it. It's all there in *Mein Kampf,* which came out in 1926, that the great empire in the East is right for dissolution. Destiny points the way. Curiously enough, Stalin never read it until the eve of the German attack on Russia in 1941. Hitler didn't try to conceal his objective or disguise his anti-Semitism.

"Now Stalin does disguise his intentions. He speaks in Marxist terms, but essentially he is creating a personal autocracy, which is not exactly in the Marxist tradition. But he never admits it. He will allow no one to speak of Stalinism. He is the exponent of Leninism. He is the realization of Marxism. He continually hammers on this, although I don't think either Lenin or Marx would have been happy with this personal autocracy, which he created. Now that of course harps back to the Czars. Stalin is 'the little father' in the Kremlin, but he can never say that openly. There's a carefully organized chorus going on all the time, saying he's the greatest ruler Russia ever had. But he presents himself as . . . the genius who realized Marxism, claiming that this is the first planned economy, the first classless society. In fact, it is a dictatorship. You can't dominate a country the size of Russia without a vast number of people accepting Stalin and his regime, but just in case they should have doubts, he institutes the purges. And Stalin never was content just to purge. The purgers themselves never knew when they too would be purged. There was a very high death rate amongst the KGB.

"Like Hitler, Stalin had no intention of allowing his power to be institutionalized. Insecurity is the essence of Stalin's rule. The evidence of this is overwhelming. As Bulganin said to Khrushchev once, 'You know, when Stalin invites you out to the dacha'—Stalin's country home—'you go, but you never know if you will come back.'

"So he's the heir to two traditions, which are totally contradictory. He claims to be the man who created the first Socialist state in the world and the head of the world Communist movement. At the same time he's the heir of the Czars. During the war, which is called the Great Patriotic War, you will find him referring to the great Czars and the great Czarist generals, Kutuzov and Suvorov. The orders and decorations, which were created for war time, were not in fact named after the socialist heroes at all. They are named after the men who defeated Napoleon. And of course Peter the Great plays a great role in Stalin's view of himself.

"So Stalin is unlike Hitler. He never tells the truth about himself. He never says, 'Look, I am the man who, while I pay lip service to Marxism, have in fact turned it inside out.' I think very possibly he would have said, 'I am the realist, the others were utopians. They thought you could do all this without using force. I know that it had to be imposed and enforced from above. That's the only way you can do it.' But he didn't say it too often. When somebody would tell him 'Comrade X's opinions are very close to yours,' he would reply "Opinions can change. I prefer fear. Fear lasts."'"

"Do you see Hitler as being like the rest of us, a bit insecure, wanting to be liked, wanting to please, or don't those motives apply?" I asked Charles Bracelen Flood.

"We have somebody who has had a very spotty record at school, who certainly is aware of the ups and downs of fortune in his own family life and in society, who's down and out in Munich and living in a shelter for homeless men for some time before the war. He gets into the war and suddenly finds this is where if you were brave and used your intelligence and collaborated with the system, the system would reward you. For the very first time in his life (he was then thirty years old), he had a medal pinned on him, compliments, not promotions, but that was because he was a part of the little staff of regimental runners at a headquarters where there wasn't that kind of rise up the ladder. Certainly he was an eccentric as well, but, yes, I think he wanted to be liked. I think he took a lot of the applause all the way through his life as some sort of substitute. He once said, 'For me, the crowd beneath is a woman' . . . to be wooed and to give him satisfaction.

"But I also think there was an astonishing kind of confidence that was with him to the end. Early in his life, at least according to boyhood friends, he was saying, 'The day will come when everyone will speak of me.' He saw the opera *Rienzi,* in which a man, based on a Roman figure, opened up a new chapter in the political life of medieval Rome, and he came out just transported, saying to his young companion, 'Yes, that'll be me. I'm going to do it.' And he later referred back to it, 'In that hour, I saw my destiny.' He was always thinking big, and I think at times he might have been terribly grateful for any recognition as he was making his way through this career as a very brave soldier in a limited but very effective capacity."

So from all we know so far about Hitler and Stalin, the question about whether they are human is really rhetorical. Of course they are. What else can they be? They were aberrations not in their humanness—for as we have seen, they were considered to be ordinary and in some respects deficient before their rise to power—but in their genius for leadership and the particular vision they pursued. It's not their humanness that is in doubt, but rather their humaneness.

They may be unique in certain ways, but they come from a long line of apocalyptic leaders—Napoleon, Genghis Khan, Julius Caesar, Ivan the Terrible, Alexander the Great—who promised to bring glory to their countries and let their followers partake in their megalomaniacal dreams. As odious as their dreams may have been, they don't disqualify them from sharing a human kinship with us or, for that matter, immunize us against someday following leaders of their ilk.

"You said that Hitler and Stalin definitely are human. From your understanding of them, do you see them as having the same kinds of feelings that most of us have—insecurities, wanting to be liked?" I asked Alan Bullock.

"They are human. But what is human? I remember Saul Bellow once said to me, 'I actually believe that the majority of people who live in Chicago are mad, clinically mad!' Of course, he's always been accused of exaggerating.

"We just don't realize what goes on behind closed doors. When I think, for instance, of the revelations of child abuse, which have opened up for us here. We knew it went on but we had no idea about the scale. I think we have a sliding scale of saints and devils. My point is that between ordinary decent people and Stalin and Hitler, it goes on in a series of gradations. They are human because, by definition, I think 'human' is so varied, it encompasses so much."

"Do you regard Hitler on the continuum of humanity?" I asked Charles Bracelen Flood.

"I think that George Will said 'He was one of us,'" he answered. "We can't get away from the fact he was indeed a human being. He was a monster, but he was one of us. I understand people's desire to say, 'Wait a minute, it doesn't take that much to be an S.S. man.' I understand that line of reasoning. I think it's a good societal, protective mechanism to say it doesn't take much to make you a bigot. [But] I feel that Hitler is totally out of the ordinary. This isn't just a man who went a little overboard. This was a man unto himself in a number of ways. . . . I don't think he understood his motivations himself. I'm not sure that anybody can really fully understand what catapulted this man onto the scene . . . what his extraordinary, energizing, demonic motivation was."

EMBRACING MYTHS IN CARICATURE

Having come to the inevitable conclusion about the humanness of these despots, we now are left with a deeper mystery. As humans, unless they were completely emotionally warped, they should have had at least a glimmering of the untold misery and suffering they caused. They must have been momentarily touched by the plight of others, either in conscious flashes of remorse or in nightmares and disturbing dreams. Surely they couldn't have been oblivious to what they had done and completely deaf to the screams of their countless victims. Whether they ever experienced pangs of guilt or had paralyzing moments of doubt about their inhumane acts, we'll never know. But if they didn't, and the evidence suggests that was so, then how did Hitler and Stalin manage to live with themselves?

The answer seems to be that they managed to do so in the same way that all humans deal with trying circumstances—by embracing certain basic myths, which allowed them to transmute adversity into good fortune, or in their case, evil into good. But with Hitler and Stalin, their personal philosopher's stone seemed even more powerful.

One of the basic myths we adopt to make our lives more palatable is the belief that we can control our lives and shape our futures more than, in fact, we do. With Hitler and Stalin, this belief assumed megalomanic proportions. They not only undertook to transform themselves—assuming names and titles that portrayed them as mythic heroes and leaders—but they tried to transform society and the world as well. Exerting almost god-like powers over the lives of others—being able to shape the morality of nations and decide whether people live or die—they lived their own lives as a symbolic denial of their relative impotency against the inexorable forces of Nature.

Then, just as all people require a purpose for living, a need for their activities to matter, Hitler and Stalin did, too. Only in their case, their purpose was an exalted one. They were embarked on a grand mission. Hitler vaguely believed that he was an agent of Providence. Stalin believed himself to be the true interpreter of Marxism and the savior of Mother Russia. Both felt they were destined to change the world and establish a new order. In these historic roles, they not only could justify whatever they did that contributed to the ultimate success of their goals but they also could attribute goodness to their deeds. Their calling transformed them from ordinary into extraordinary beings and also gave purpose to their lives.

Next, we've noted the importance of the love bond for a stable sense of self. Hitler and Stalin also showed their need for this love bond in their relationship to intimates and society as a whole. They strove to develop love and devotion from their subordinates, as well as adulation by society as a whole, if not by their charisma and deeds, then through propaganda, intimidation, and fear. To some extent, they seemed capable of caring for others, but only when these others conformed to certain prescribed roles, such as a loving mother, a dutiful wife, a devoted daughter, or a compliant friend, but never on the basis of mutual equality or on a meaningful psychological level. Their love was abstract and remote, confined mostly to the bond between themselves and the person-in-the-role rather than to the particular person. They showed this *par excellence* on a broader scale in their avowed love for the common people, the *volk* or the *proletariat*, and in their desire to be admired by them.

They also displayed the same need to perpetuate their self that most humans do. Their judge was not God or mankind, but history itself. Hitler created the Third Reich, and Stalin helped to create the first socialist state, creations which they believed would live on long beyond their deaths. To their minds, a utopian society possessed an inherent permanence, if not in reality, then at least in recorded history. To insure that history would remember them as they wanted to be remembered, Stalin actually rewrote history, page by page, and his place in it, and Hitler deliberately cultivated his legendary status and commissioned grand architectural monuments and art to commemorate his reign.

Lastly, in their quest for immortality, with only rare exceptions, they viewed their victims as abstractions (e.g., kulaks, misfits, Jews, gypsies), who only existed generically as statistics or collectively as members of despised groups and not as distinct individuals. Shylock's lament, "If you prick us, do we not bleed? If you tickle us, do we not laugh? If you poison us, do we not die? And if you wrong us, shall we not seek revenge?" falls on deaf ears. People existed, even their loyal minions, only as entities who could help them realize their apocalyptic vision or as impediments who stood in the way.

All of these observations, then, suggest how Hitler and Stalin managed to live with themselves. But there is another side to the equation. These men could not have committed their horrendous crimes without the active complicity of many of their countrymen. What also calls for explanation is how seemingly decent people with more modest personal goals could implement the policies of their evil leaders and reconcile what they did with their moral systems and their personal sense of self. It explains nothing to say that entire nations were temporarily insane or duped by their leaders or were completely ignorant of what was going on.

HEALERS OR KILLERS?

Between 1939 and 1945 the Nazis systematically murdered about two hundred thousand mentally ill or physically handicapped people under the banner of euthanasia, people whom they saw as "life unworthy of life." In the interests of racial fitness, many psychiatrists not only supported the compulsory sterilization of mental patients but adopted the Nazi policy of killing retarded children and chronic mental cases by gassing, starvation, and lethal injections. In his book, *Death and Deliverance*, Michael Burleigh examines how members of the health establishment, sometimes along with the tacit approval of the relatives of these patients themselves, could have participated in this program.[6] His conclusions are sobering.

It appears that once certain conditions exist, people can justify even the most egregious crimes. We start with the economic factor, which always seems capable of getting people's attention. The asylums were overcrowded and regarded as a financial drain on society, especially at a time when Germany was mobilizing for war. This got people worrying about the potential impact of this on their own buying power and savings. We add the spreading philosophy of social Darwinism—survival of the fittest and the need to purify the race—that the National Socialist government was promulgating. Here was a pseudoscientific rationale that held intellectual appeal. Then we add the "Führer principle," which meant abdicating personal responsibility for one's actions by recognizing the immediate authority of the regional health officials, who were acting as agents of Hitler.

To make the sterilization or killing of emotionally ill and mentally retarded patients more palatable, the Racial and Political Office of the National Socialist Party orchestrated a propaganda campaign through films and other public media to criminalize, degrade, and dehumanize these individuals. These patients were depicted as "creatures," "existences," "idiots," "degenerates," "obscene beings," and "subhumans," and as a terrible burden to the German worker and as a potential source of racial pollution. In one film, for instance, the audience was informed that in the last seventy years the population of the country had increased by 50 percent, while in the same period the number of hereditarily ill had risen by 450 percent. "If this development continues, in fifty years there would be one hereditarily ill person for every four healthy people," the narrator claimed. "An endless column of horror would march into the nation. The Law for the Prevention of Hereditarily Diseased Progeny is not interference in divine law, but rather the restoration of natural order which mankind has disrupted because of a false sense of humanity."[7]

Operating in this climate, those involved in the euthanasia program seemed convinced that they were engaged in almost a divine mission. It's no surprise then to find after the war, when many of them came to trial, that they should have justified their actions. Listen to this account.

"The life of the insane person has, for himself and his relatives, lost all purpose, and consists only of pain and misery. . . . This means the doctor . . . particularly in view of the person's spiritual life—[has the] duty to free the person from his unworthy condition, so—I might even say—from his prison."[8]

Here is an even more righteous justification. "I do not feel that I am incriminated. I was motivated by absolutely humane feelings. I never had any other belief than that . . . the painful lives of these [poor miserable] creatures were to be shortened. The only thing I regret . . . is pain was inflicted on the relatives. But I am convinced that these relatives have overcome this sorrow today and that they themselves feel that their dead relatives were freed from suffering."[9]

So it seems that under the right conditions, with certain beliefs and the approval of society, the killers and murderers of thousands can portray themselves as humanitarians and dedicated to relieving human suffering. Depending on whether we view others as human, saints can become sinners or sinners can become saints.

How can these individuals believe something so blatantly untrue? The reasons they can do so aren't so different from the reasons we can embrace certain beliefs in our own personal life stories. Capitalizing on people's needs, fears, and concerns, as well as their desire for social approval, the German and Russian leaders promulgated a seemingly plausible ideology that met all the criteria for a good therapeutic narrative and fit in with people's attraction for certain myths. It offered people the chance to participate in a grand cultural drama, in which they could be on the side of good. They were exposed to a world view that offered simple explanations for their concerns and simple solutions for their cure. They were able to bolster their beliefs with pseudoscientific arguments about race or economics or the historical process or fabricated evidence offered by those in authority. Add to these ingredients the predisposition of many people to believe what they were told about Jews, gypsies, or kulaks—whom they already were suspicious of or envied—and it was little wonder that substantial numbers of people readily adopted the rationales offered for war and the persecution of certain groups. As for those who continued to harbor doubts about the prevalent political views, their desire to participate in this grand drama and their fear of being punished or killed if they didn't were often sufficient for many of them to suspend their critical faculties and become converts to the cause.

Perhaps one of the most unsettling issues in the understanding of evil is how intelligent, cultured physicians, who take an oath to preserve life and relieve suffering, could become the agents of pain and death. In a remarkable study, Robert Jay Lifton interviewed twenty-eight Nazi physicians who played varying roles in implementing Hitler's Final Solution.[10] At the concentration camp at Auschwitz, certain of these doctors selected who would live, supervised the killings in the gas chambers, ordered and oversaw the killing of debilitated patients, the mentally ill, and the retarded (with phenol injections into their hearts and other methods), and performed forced sterilizations and dangerous experimentations on gypsies, Jews, and other undesirables.

The question is how could they engage in this horrific behavior that seemed to violate everything they valued and stood for? According to Lifton, they did this through certain complex mental maneuvers. One of the most important maneuvers was to adopt a rationale that could justify their action. What could justify their actions, even make them worthy, was to view themselves as biological soldiers who were acting in accord with natural history and the biology of man. Along with this view was the Nazi notion that killing was a difficult but necessary form of personal ideal, a type of self-sacrifice for the good of the nation. Through euthanasia and sterilization, they could help cure society of its sickness and help purify the Aryan race.

The kind of psychological adjustment they had to make to accommodate these views largely involved "doubling," a division of the self into two functioning wholes so that a part-self acts as the entire self. The process of doubling, which bears resemblances to dissociation, the mental mechanism underlying multiple personality, let them maintain a concentration-camp self that could function in so diabolical a setting and an ordinary self that represented a humane physician, husband, and father. The doctors then could view their concentration-camp selves as a form of psychological survival in a death-oriented setting and not have to give up their basic views of themselves.

To maintain this concentration camp self without guilt, these physicians had to resort to mental gymnastics. Convinced that what they were doing was medically and ethically justifiable, they found ways to kill without killing by regarding their victims as less than human or even as vermin, a social infestation that had to be cured. Besides, the Jews brought this on themselves, they reasoned, and therefore deserved what they got. Those who couldn't accept this rationale had access to other mental defenses, such as splitting or distancing, which allowed a kind of psychic numbing and derealization. Yet there is another often overlooked factor that underlies all these mental maneuvers, which is the force of daily routine. Working everyday in the extreme conditions of a concentration camp deconstructs the broader values people have, and after a while nothing seems strange. People come to find meaning in their daily tasks rather in the nature of those tasks.

The power of duty and daily routine to supply meaning for people takes on a chilling importance when we examine the activities of Adolf Eichmann, the person charged with carrying out the Final Solution. What manner of person was this who could take professional pride in how many people he put to death and how efficiently he did so? According to the psychiatrists who examined him during his trial, the answer was that he was normal, even exceptionally so. From his report, he insisted that he held no special animosity toward the millions of people he put to death. He was a patriotic bureaucrat who simply was doing his duty. Like any conscientious administrator, he wanted to do his job well. Hannah Arendt, commenting on Eichmann's role in the Holocaust, along with those of many others like him, characterized it as the "banality of evil."[11]

I asked Alan Bullock whether the banality of evil explained any of Hitler's or Stalin's behavior.

He pointed out that neither Hitler nor Stalin put anybody to death or observed any of these scenes. "They wanted to know what went on. Hitler wanted photographs, but he didn't go to see. He didn't take part in it. It's a very interesting question, a terrible question. When do you last think Hitler saw a Jew? A very long time before he started to exterminate them. So they had become an abstraction in his mind.

"Stalin actually destroyed people he knew very well indeed, people who had been closest to him after Lenin. Trotsky's an example. There were many others. But I don't think Hannah Arendt is talking about Hitler or Stalin. If you use this phrase as I think she was using it, it applies to the bureaucrats of terror and murder. In the death camps, the extermination camps, Himmler ran two alternatives. You could either work the Jews to death if they were strong enough or you could gas them. And with every train that came in, the doctors picked out those who looked strong enough to put into the armament works because they were desperately short of labor. They were very short-handed with six to seven million foreign laborers, and they could work these people to death, literally.

"But the S.S. accountants worked out the comparative cost-benefit of this exercise. 'If you keep these Jews alive you have to feed them and house them while they do their work, whereas you don't spend anything on them if you gas them.' They actually boast that they have raised the productivity of death. That is to say, they've killed more men, children, and women in relation to what they have invested in building the camps and paying the wages of the people who do it. That to me has a particular horror. It's the dehumanizing of it.

"When I was working on Hitler, I remember coming across an exchange of correspondence between the S.S. central office in Berlin and the S.S. in Russia, who were at that time killing people by pushing them into vans and coupling up the hose and gassing them. Here is a quote from one of the letters: 'We need to know a lot more before we can agree to your demand for extra rubber hoses. How is it that these are worn out so quickly? They shouldn't be.' So back comes the answer with 'Your reference, My reference' at the top of the letter. 'Well, we have our problems. We've been trying to do this quickly, and the men don't like it because they want to be off on Saturday afternoons and Sundays, and particularly if there are any football matches. They play games with the soldiers. They have a team. The fact is if you put them to work on Saturdays, they rush the stuff, and they push them through at a fast rate, and just abuse the process. We find it very difficult to stamp this out because the demand is coming for more and more. We haven't got enough help to deal with all the Jews you find.'

"That all belongs with banality. The only time Himmler ever saw any of this he fainted. But then he said to his S.S. officers: 'You have to nerve yourself. This is one of the greatest pages in our history. You have to do these things, which you and I don't like. But you know that you do this for the future of the German people. This is one of the glorious pages of our history that may never be written because it has to be kept secret.'"

Charles Bracelen Flood took a somewhat different perspective on the issue of banality.

"Hitler was banal only in the fact that when he was sipping beer in a beer garden with some of his early Nazi party cronies, he could be just another Munich burgher sitting there. But I think he's a psychopath. I know that's rather an old fashioned term, but I don't see anything banal about a man who was quoted as saying, well into the time of the Holocaust, 'Thank God, I've always avoided persecuting my enemies.' That to me is such overwhelming evidence of somebody who is not in touch with reality."

What this also points up is how the deconstruction of an evil act can rid it of its overall meaning.[12] By breaking down a complex activity into a series of component parts, each of which seems mundane and trivial, the causal connections among them loosen and the responsibility for what later happens disappears. In this manner, the meaning associated with the whole becomes transferred to each of its parts. A doctor, for instance, can decide which new prisoner is physically fit for hard labor in the concentration camp and which isn't without having to see his act as imposing an immediate death sentence on the rejects. All he is doing, he reasons with himself, is making a medical judgment.

Flood's observation about Hitler's psychopathic tendencies bears special mention. There are certain people who are so biologically and psychologically constituted that they deconstruct actions almost as soon as they engage in them. With psychopaths, for instance, the moment is all that counts. Primed to respond impulsively to satisfy their immediate needs and wants, they aren't likely to associate a deed with its potential long term consequences. They regard people as objects, whom they can manipulate and use. They show no compunction about causing others harm not only because they lack empathy for others' plight, but also because their own needs and pleasures are paramount.

Though it takes a special evil genius to become a Hitler, the issue is whether all of us have the potential to be Nazis, and even more to the point, to participate in genocide. From Lifton's studies, almost anybody has that potential under certain conditions. It isn't my intention to comment on the many instances of cruel and inhuman behavior by ordinary people at different times in history, motivated by ethnic, religious, or ideological differences, or simply by greed and a thirst for power. This is irrelevant for our purposes. What is relevant is that this potential exists, and for it to be realized, certain adjustments in the self-concept need to be made.

Obviously, one adjustment that people who engage in evil make is that they don't see what they are doing as evil. Evil is what others do, people different from them, the enemy. And if they themselves do it, then they weren't themselves. Some external agency made them do so. Or some aberrant force within them was responsible. Or they did so in a fit of passion or insanity. Or what they did stemmed from a noble purpose. The point is that their real self wouldn't be capable of a heinous crime, or so they prefer to believe.

The ways that ordinary people can be induced to engage in sadistic or cruel behavior has been documented in the classic study by Stanley Milgram.[13] The basic paradigm of the study was to tell participants that they were helping to test the effects of punishment on learning, but unbeknownst to them, the real aim was to test the extent to which they would comply with the experimenter's instructions to inflict pain on others. Sitting before an impressive shock generator, participants were required to administer shocks of increasing severity, ranging from fifteen volts to 450 volts, to the "learner," who had electrodes placed on him. The designations of these shock levels varied from "Slight Shock" to "Danger—Severe Shock." The participants, however, didn't know that the learner, or victim, actually was an actor, and the shocks he would receive to help him learn weren't real.

As the participants increased the intensity of shock during the session, the "victim" feigned increasing discomfort, protesting as the shocks escalated, and at 285 volts pleading and letting out an agonizing scream. When the subjects began hesitating or showing moral qualms about increasing the shock, the experimenter, representing a legitimate authority, ordered them to continue.

The results of the study were startling. Almost two-thirds of the participants, who were drawn from the working, managerial, and professional classes, were classified as "obedient," continuing to shock the victim no matter how painful the shocks seemed to be. Trying to fathom the motives of the participants, Milgram identified a number of factors, the most important of which were the adjustments they made in their thinking that kept them from disobeying the authority when he insisted they inflict more pain. One of their adjustments, for example, was to become so absorbed in the technical aspects of the task that they lost sight of its broader consequences. This fragmentation of behavior, divorced from its overall context, was reminiscent of the actions of the petty functionaries in the concentration camps. Also, wanting to put on a competent performance, they entrusted the morality of the situation to the authority they were serving. The obedient subjects also saw themselves as not responsible for their actions. Like the many concentration camp guards who claimed they were just "doing their duty," when the experimenter told them, "The experiment requires that you continue," they deferred to this higher moral authority and justified what they did as being motivated by the pursuit of scientific truth. Then, once having obeyed the authority, many participants found it convenient to see the victim as unworthy, whose punishment was justified because of his own deficiencies, or in other experiments, in which they were collaborators, to shift the responsibility to the person who pulled the switch. Even when some subjects protested that the commands of the experimenter were morally wrong, they still acceded to them because they couldn't bring themselves to make an open break with authority. In other words, we find the same psychological forces at work in the vast majority of "normal" experimental subjects as we do in those who actually perpetrated evil.

BEARING WITNESS

So far we've examined how people handle evil in themselves. We haven't looked at how they handle it in others. Generally, what we do with others is what we do for ourselves if these others are part of our extended sense of self. Depending on the circumstances, our self systems include our lovers, our children, our families, our peers, members of our race, gender, or religion, and our countrymen. We seek to exonerate them from blame because we identify with them and their guilt reflects on us. We stand by our spouses, finding excuses for their immoral behavior, because we know them as people who aren't basically bad or because, over the years, we have slowly absorbed some of their value systems. We excuse the excesses of our countrymen during war because they only got carried away in defending our national interests. Or we excuse the actions of our comrades who adhere to the same causes, even with absurd reasons. Listen, for example, to the excuse a right-to-life minister made for Paul Hill, a former minister himself, who killed an abortion clinic doctor and his volunteer escort in Pensacola, Florida. "He believes strongly that if he is executed, or only sentenced to life imprisonment, he will have made a statement as to his very strong belief in *the sanctity of human life to Almighty God* [emphasis mine]."[14]

Now what about those people, namely biographers, who sometimes have the task of bringing psychologically destructive or even murderous people to life but who only can do so by also portraying their humanness? This is a intriguing issue, since as certain of my biographers have informed me, empathy with their subjects is essential for understanding them, and it's even better if they like and admire them, especially when they sometimes spend years absorbed by their lives. I was especially interested to learn how decent and intelligent people, who stared evil straight in the eye, managed to remain decent and objective in response. This is so for the biographers of such evil geniuses as Hitler or Stalin. It's perhaps even more so for the person who interviewed the Nazi doctors.

In his chapter on "bearing witness," Robert Jay Lifton mentioned the psychological strain on him of sitting in the room with Nazi doctors while his mind conjured up images of Jews lined up for selection at Auschwitz and mental patients being gassed at killing centers. To conduct his research, he concluded that he would have to view these medical perpetrators, whatever their relationship to evil, "as human beings and nothing else." In his words: "That meant requiring of myself a form of empathy for Nazi doctors: I had to imagine my way into their situation, not to exonerate but to seek knowledge of human susceptibility to evil. The logic of my position was clear enough: only a measure of empathy, however reservedly offered, could help one grasp the psychological components of the *anti-empathic* evil in which many of these Nazi doctors had engaged."[15] He had to do this, knowing all the while that these same doctors had directed their murderous activities at "my own people, at me."

To cope with this impossible situation, Lifton said he had to alter his sense of self sufficiently to join the doctor in his Nazi world. At the same time, he had to remember the victims involved, hold onto an ethical content consistent with his own sense of self, and then justify the empathy he showed during this psychological juggling act. Yet what Lifton doesn't say, and what we only can read between the lines, is that he uses many of the same mental mechanisms to gather his materials as his subjects used in their work. He psychologically went about his distasteful daily tasks of interviewing these Nazi doctors in a way similar to the way that they went about theirs: justifying what he was doing as serving a broader scientific and social purpose, and treating his subjects as somewhat less than people. They were humans, yes, but they were odious creatures nonetheless, and as research subjects, they served as laboratory rats of sorts. To continue his work, Lifton had to resort to a form of "doubling" as well, distinguishing between what the scientific part of his personality was willing to do and what the human part of him believed. None of my observations should be construed as in any way critical of Lifton. What he did was heroic and represents a definite contribution to our understanding of the nature of evil. What he also did, though perhaps unwittingly, was to show that the psychological gulf separating the perpetrator of a heinous deed and someone who bears witness to it isn't as wide as it may seem, at least in the ways of dealing with the presence of evil.

That the investigator of evil and the perpetrator of evil exist on the same human continuum and have access to similar mental mechanisms for dealing with the evil is well illustrated in the personal account of how Robert C. Tucker, a biographer of Joseph Stalin, responded to the evil of his subject. Aware that Stalin had no consciousness of his own villainy, Tucker, in an effort to reenact and understand his subject's mind, tried to reconcile Stalin's duplicities and atrocities with his inner picture of himself as a righteous man and noble ruler. "This takes a bit of doing," Tucker explained, "but the whole meaning and worth of the scholarly enterprise rests upon it."[16] However, because of his intense negative feelings toward Stalin, Tucker was upset that certain members of Stalin's inner circle failed to assassinate him when they had a chance to do so. "They must have known," Tucker wrote, "that Stalin, like a mad dog, had to be destroyed." Then he went on to confess: "Sometime in the quiet of my study, I must have found myself bursting out to their ghosts: 'For God's sake, stab him with a knife, or pick up a heavy object and bash his brains out, for the lives you save may include your own!'"[17] He was shaken enough by his own murderous impulses toward Stalin, which a colleague observed was the voice of Stalin in him, to wonder whether that disqualified him from writing an objective biography about his subject. But he put aside this objection. Rationalizing, he claimed that when trying to puzzle out the behavior of an infinitely evil person, "one's inquisitiveness, the urge to illuminate what went on inside the man that led him to act as he did, the need to explain to oneself as well as others, to comprehend and communicate things that may have evaded understanding, can become a dominating drive, and this drive can counteract the simplifying mental tendencies that hatred of the subject may generate."[18] This "passion for curiosity" is not so different from what Lifton experienced when working with the Nazi doctors. It seems to derive from the common mental defense mechanism of "intellectualization," which lets us separate and suppress disturbing feelings from our intellectual activity. It's often the way that I myself react in my work toward people who have committed heinous deeds, and, I confess, toward certain bigoted, hate-filled patients I don't like.

"The question is, have you gotten any criticism for taking these individuals on as a kind of historical biography," I asked Alan Bullock. "I've talked to some other biographers who have talked about the importance of having empathy for their subjects as a way of getting into their heads and trying to understand the way they see things. I wondered whether that issue has been raised, and what you think about dealing with characters that you actually might loathe."

"I find it a very difficult question to answer," he responded. "I am suspicious of the word 'empathy' because it's pretty difficult to get inside somebody else's head. Great dramatists, like Shakespeare, have that power. I don't think I have.

"I honestly don't know why I was ever drawn to this as a question. To me, it's a series of coincidences and opportunities. Somebody asked me to write a book on Hitler. I spent the war finding out a great deal about Nazi Germany. So it fitted perfectly, and the book was a success. After I retired from running a college twenty-five years later, I wanted to prove to myself that I could still do this. My second book on Hitler was written in my seventies. I was seventy when I began and I'm seventy-eight now. I wanted to write another book about history just to show I was a historian, one last go. And then I hit on the idea of comparing Hitler and Stalin. Now, any psychiatrist would say, 'My dear chap, your capacity for self-deception is extraordinary. Don't you know that this is because. . . .' But I can't psychoanalyze myself, so I don't really know why I have done this book. One of the things I think that happens is whenever you get into something like this, you become fascinated by the chase. You become fascinated by the actual process of finding the documents, of tracking them down, and saying 'Yes, I see, that's how it fits together.' Now I wouldn't go so far as to say that means I got inside Hitler, but I can see how Hitler at the time wanted the Nazi/Soviet Pact and I can see how, for opposite reasons, Stalin wanted it. Now that clicked, and I remember the intellectual satisfaction of seeing how these actions fitted together. Whether I can understand motivation. . . . I mean there's the famous story told by one of Stalin's people, who had been with him one evening quite early on in his career. Someone asked, 'What's the greatest pleasure in life, the victory in the end?' Stalin said, 'I think the greatest pleasure in life is to find somebody who is a bastard, fix it so he's finished, and then go home to bed and sleep soundly.' Now I don't understand that. Hitler and Stalin are two very difficult people to empathize with. I think I anesthetized myself to some degree. There were days, however, when the horror of it all came home to me. Curiously enough, after I finished this second book, I was in Austria just over a year ago, and was in a house that somebody had lent us, and for some reason I never found out, that house had an atmosphere of evil in it. I had to leave. I couldn't stay in it. This was a perfectly ordinary, modest farmer's house, no associations that I knew, but there came over me the sense of horror at what I had been writing about.

"Most of the time, however, I think I anesthetized myself. That would be the honest answer. But I am deeply troubled by the question."

"My reaction was not one of empathy," Charles Bracelen Flood informed me, in response to my question about the importance of this quality for a biographer. "To know Hitler was to despise him. At the same time I was deeply impressed with his abilities, with the understanding that these abilities were used for evil ends. He was not in any way a caricature figure as I encountered him. As he grew in my mind, I was constantly impressed by his ability. In fact, I often thought, 'If only this degree of intelligence and energy could have been harnessed to good ends in that terrible postwar situation in Germany, what a contribution this man might have been able to make.'

TELLING GOOD AND EVIL APART

Of course, in an ultimate philosophical sense, all of this discussion may be moot if we hold there is no such thing as evil. As Hitler himself argued, conscience is an invention of the weak, a way to keep the strong in check. Social Darwinism is the ultimate measure. As abhorrent as this notion is, humans throughout history have shown again and again through their actions that they embrace it, regardless of the rationales they offer. What some define as terrorism, others see as heroism. What some define as liberation, others see as oppression. What some define as aggression, others see as self-defense. What some define as holy wars, others see as slaughter and carnage. What some define as justifiable, others see as inexcusable. Unless we adopt an absolute morality—you shouldn't kill, torture, or make any human being suffer under any conditions—we risk having evil construed by certain others as good and making all standards of behavior relative.

So that we not become too confused by these contradictory notions about what constitutes evil, legal and moral authorities instruct us how to tell good and evil apart. Killing, for example, is generally bad, but it's good when done on behalf of our country, while upholding the law, in self-defense, or for the punishment of a crime. It's potentially excusable (or at least understandable) when done in the heat of passion or in response to sexual or physical abuse. Judgment is placed on hold when the person is insane at the time of the murder. What is inexcusable is a crime that is planned and deliberate, which isn't sanctioned socially and deviates from prevalent mores.

When evil is perpetrated under the aegis of society, it must be transformed into good by having it serve some noble purpose: to preserve democracy, for the glory of God, for "ethnic cleansing," or in Nazi Germany's case, to purify the race. One of the most effective ways to eliminate guilt is to portray our victims as less than human—as savages, infidels, heretics, nonbelievers, degenerates, or as abominations—or as a direct threat to our families, our way of life, our country, and therefore, us. When other people are seen as subhuman, torture, mayhem, murder, and slaughter aren't necessarily evil, but may be construed as necessary actions to promote a greater good.

Aside from our need to be in tune with our surrounding culture, our self-system needs to be in tune with itself. For the story of our life to flow smoothly, our actions and thoughts need to be compatible with our basic assumptions about the world and our purpose in being. The actions and thoughts we regard as evil interrupt the narrative flow of our life story, and if they can't be comfortably incorporated into it, lead to a destabilization of the self. When we can't accept parts of ourselves as belonging to us, we maneuver to disassociate ourselves from them by splitting, doubling, and walling them off, or by creating multiple selves. And if these maneuvers don't work, we become progressively immobilized psychologically.

These observations about how people deal with evil—whether Hitler, Stalin, their followers, or ourselves—reveal a fundamental truth about the way our self-systems are constituted. The construction of our self-system is based less on a reliance on truth and goodness than on the need to preserve inner harmony. Our self-system serves us best when discordances and incompatibilities can be put aside so that it can deal optimally with day to day events or with any external circumstances that threaten our survival. The acceptance of stark reality isn't the primary concern of the self-system: adaptiveness and optimal functioning are. To achieve this, the self must reconcile our thoughts, feelings, and actions with socially approved motives. What experiences it can't comfortably incorporate, assimilate, or integrate within itself to promote inner harmony, it extrudes, walls off, or projects onto some external agency. It may even resort to ingenious but convoluted strategies, as evidenced, for example, by those who claim that an evil like the Holocaust never existed and was a fiction perpetrated by its victims.

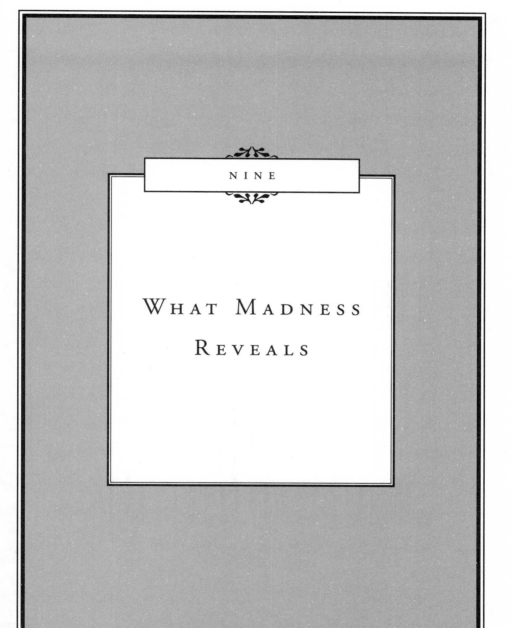

NINE

WHAT MADNESS
REVEALS

PLATO BELIEVED THAT A POET'S INSPIRATION WAS FUELED in moments of "divine madness," and William James, a dominant figure in American psychology, wondered whether a body temperature of 103° or 104° Fahrenheit might be more conducive to the creative spirit than the usual 98°F. In more recent times, others have claimed that mind-altering drugs such as LSD, could allow people to explore different dimensions of their selves, by escaping the strictures of social mores and conventions.[1]

These observations about the potential value of madness, delirium, or intoxication are intriguing, but they shouldn't be misconstrued. No doubt, abnormalities in brain function can teach us much about the nature of reality, particularly how subjective and relative it is, but they offer no insights about what is really "real." No matter how compelling or transcendent their experiences, deranged persons don't necessarily see reality more accurately than sane ones. They simply see it differently.

SANITY AS A MENTAL STRAITJACKET

It's possible to argue, as some have done, that sanity is only a socially approved form of madness. We go about our daily business—involved in our work, taking pleasure in our loved ones, and planning for the future—trying not to dwell on our inevitable death, the eventual loss of all those we care for, and the possibility that all our beliefs are false. To deal with the potential meaninglessness of our predicament, we engage in an array of mental maneuvers that make ignorance seem like truth, that shield us from the stark reality of our predicament, and that let us have fervent beliefs with no basis in fact. Without conscious awareness, we repress emotionally painful experiences, project our own unwanted intentions onto others, rationalize our behaviors, deny whatever feelings we don't want to accept, or sublimate any taboo urges. With a perceptual apparatus limited to only five senses, which only can transduce sensory signals from our physical environment and body in certain prescribed ways, and with a limited mental capacity of about ten billion neurons to process all the information that passes through our brains, and with only certain socially sanctioned ways available to interpret this information, and with only limited ways to act on it and shape our immediate environment, we move about "sanely" in a world that is distorted by our cerebral deficiencies and cognitive limitations.

However, since we are communal creatures, we need to be able to interpret our experiences and communicate our needs using shared symbols. To insure a common reality, our parents, siblings, friends, teachers, and preachers teach us while we are growing up what information is important, how to interpret it, and how to communicate it. Sanity represents social consensus, a general agreement that what we perceive is what others perceive, too. This "politics of experience," to use a term coined by R. D. Laing, is essential not only for us to function smoothly in society but also for society to exist.[2] Sanity becomes the lingua franca for social existence. Unless we share certain fundamental assumptions about reality with others, we are apt to see them as mad.

Given the impermanence of our existence and the eventual death of all our loved ones, we can argue that depression and anxiety represent the only "sane" response to this scary situation, and that being cheerful and remaining oblivious to this reality is really insane. Louise DeSalvo interprets much of Virginia Woolf's seemingly irrational behavior in this way, not as psychopathology but as an adaptive response to her past sexual abuse and the circumstances of her life.

"I see her as grappling heroically over the course of her life," she told me, "with trying to figure out why she is embattled, why she is depressed, why she feels she is fragmented, why she feels a sense of pride eludes her. I see a person grappling with the issue of a fragmented self as essentially healthy, not as unhealthy. Given the fact that Woolf was grappling with these issues in the context of a society that did not understand that an incest survivor very often feels depressed, with a sense of futility or self-worthlessness, I see her life-long dialectic with her own troubled self as essentially that of a wholesome person in pursuit of trying to get some very real answers to issues that were important for her."

MADNESS AS A NATURAL EXPERIMENT

What would losing your mind, going mad, do to your sense of self? How would you respond when thinking rationally became difficult, when you no longer could trust your perceptions, when you began suspecting people of plotting against you, when your reality props dissolved and almost everything you previously took for granted now started to seem unreal? What adjustments would you have to make in your self-concept to accommodate all these strange things happening to you? Luckily, we have access to personal accounts of people who went through such experiences to learn what they tell us about the nature of the self.

By examining the impact of different forms of mental illness on our minds, we can identify different aspects of the self and establish what their functions are. Just as the many kinds of brain injuries caused by war, disease, or surgical lesions let scientists map out the functions of affected parts of the brain, the various forms of mental illness likewise let us tease apart the different functions of the self. When a part of the mind isn't operating properly, we not only find defective functioning by certain components within the self-system but overcompensation by other components as well.

The lessons that madness can teach us about the self come from mental aberrations in their broadest sense—neurophysiological disturbances, drugs, obsessive-compulsive conditions, depression, mania, dissociative states, panic disorders, and schizophrenia—which have either pathological or natural causes. All mental aberrations needn't be psychotic. When we dissect out their differential impact on the self, the composite picture that emerges reveals certain aspects of the self-system that are ordinarily masked by "normal" brain states.

THE SENSE OF "I"

The sense of "I" stems from our being aware, along with our capacity to observe, decide, and reflect. Because it is closely bound to memory, it's responsible for the sense of continuity and progression of our experiences, the sense of constancy of our perceptions, and the sense of owning our experiences. This part of our self-system exists from an early age and continues throughout our entire adult lives without noticeable change. It is a basic property of normal brain functioning that lets us be conscious of ourselves, even though it has no identity of its own.

Disturbances in our sense of "I" become apparent during conditions that profoundly alter consciousness. For example, in a series of radical self-experiments, John C. Lilly, a scientist who is perhaps best known for his research on communications between dolphins and humans, explored his own consciousness after taking high doses of LSD while floating suspended in a tank of water under conditions of sensory deprivation.[3] Achieving what he called a "supraself" level that, at its ultimate, represented a fusion with the universal mind, Lilly made two conclusions during his inner explorations that kept his fear of going crazy in check. One was that his body could take care of itself when he left it, and the other was that he always could return to his body if he found it "too tough out there." During his mental trips, a "self-metaprogrammer" let him be aware of his own mental processes as long as his emotions weren't too intense. When that happened, the activities of this "I" faded and other systems ran his mental bio-computer. Being literally "out of his mind" was not sufficient to eliminate the monitoring activities of the "I," which only became submerged under the swelling tides of emotion.

My own experience with LSD, while not taken under such extreme conditions, mirrors certain of Lilly's observations about the self. While being monitored by a colleague after ingesting fifty micrograms of d-lysergic acid diethylamide, I found myself continuously commenting on myself as I drifted around in a world of fantastic colors and delicious sensations. Although I claimed no need to communicate my experiences, my voice kept reporting on my subjective experiences as though it was some distant commentator that was scrutinizing me. I kept my eyes half closed, noticing beautiful and magnificent yellows and oranges, which took on a great personal significance. The colors, which kept changing on the firmament of my mind, became my world, and I began blending and mixing with them, and I was prepared to do so forever.

What I learned from my experience with LSD was that my sense of "I" and sense of "me" could be teased apart, with the "I" becoming a relatively dispassionate spectator and commentator on the experiences and activities of the "me." While this happened, the ordinary boundaries I ascribed to my self began to dis-

appear, and I could blend into and become one with the objects of my perceptions. I could see what I heard, feel what I saw, and taste what I smelled within
a timeless and spaceless universe. All the while, my "I" automatically gave a running, often fragmented, choppy mental commentary about what was transpiring,
only ceasing when my experiences became very intense.

What my experience also taught me was that this inner "I," this beam of subvocal awareness, could treat my thoughts, feelings, and perceptions with the
same clinical dispassion as it could the colleague who was monitoring me or
other objects in the room. My body and its experiences were part of me, yet they
weren't. Liberated from the artificial bounds of my body, my awareness not only
flooded the room but also encompassed the universe. Outside my corporeal
prison, I could experience cosmic consciousness. There was no future and no
past. The present was eternity. All that existed was an almost pure awareness,
tainted by an inner commentator that felt obliged, like a talkative child driving
in the rear seat of a car, to point out everything along the roadside.

A heightened sense of "I" not only comes from out-of-body experiences. As
it happens, the more the observing and commenting "I" casts its spotlight on our
experiences and activities, the more disconnected we are apt to feel. In *The Eden
Express*, Mark Vonnegut, the son of the famous novelist, documented the dis-
mantling of his self and the autonomous operation of an inner executor as he
progressed into a schizophrenic-like psychosis. "I felt no lack of energy, in fact I
had a supersurplus; but my hands, arms, and legs were getting all confused. I'd
get all hung up on how perfectly beautiful one muscle was, exactly what it did,
and get it to do it just right. But then all the others would go off on their own
little trip. I was losing my coordination as well as my concentration. . . . It was
like something in me knew I would be unable to function, and got me ready by
telling me ahead of time that it didn't matter."[4]   Then other indications of reality, previously taken for granted by Vonnegut, also went awry. As happened with
me under LSD, he also stopped experiencing time as being continuous. Sometimes when he came back from his cosmic jaunts, he felt like no time had passed
in his absence even though it seemed that he crammed a year or more into an
instant of everyone else's time. At other times when he came back to reality, he
felt that he had been in a state of suspended animation, with years passing for
everybody but him.

The existence of hallucinations, another important feature of psychosis, offers us other insights about the operations of this sense of "I." Lori Schiller, in *The Quiet Room*, gives a vivid account of her experience with the hallucinating voices that constantly cursed and reviled her and told her, "You must die." These voices were with her when she awoke, when she got dressed, when she ate. They were with her when she sat in the hospital dayroom, trying to think of something to do. They even intruded into her sleep, sometimes yelling so loudly that they woke her up, leaving her shaking and frightened.

"The closest I ever got to a friendly Voice was that of the Narrator," she wrote. "He described my actions instant by instant, not leaving out even the tiniest, most insignificant thing. A hundred times a day, he commented on my movements.

"'She is now walking through the door,' the Narrator said. 'She's wiping her feet, little ass. Wiping her feet on the rug in the entryway. She's going into the kitchen. Ha! Ha! You fat piece of lard, of lard. Go to hell. Ha! Ha! You look sad. You look like shit. You are shit. She's now walking into the day room. She's going to turn down the TV set. To die, asshole. Ha! Ha! Ha! . . .'

"The Narrator taunted me, made fun of me. Sometimes even threatened me a little. But mostly he just talked about what I was doing. And his manner was less intrusive, his Voice level less loud, and his overall demeanor less scary than the others. I didn't fear him as much as I feared the others. I just wanted his annoying banter to go away.

"Sometimes I heard one Voice laughing, a single witchlike Voice that screeched and cackled in derision. Sometimes that Voice would be joined by a second, and then a third. Sometimes they chanted the same thing over and over again, like Voices rehearsing for a play.

"'To die!' they charged. 'To die!' I must have heard that a thousand times a day."[5]

What this account illustrates so well is that even within the "I" component of the self-system, when the disruption is great enough, we can tease apart an overall sense of awareness, an observer function, from a narrating component, although they mostly operate in unison. The more the observer becomes aware of the narrator, the more the narrator takes on the qualities of a hallucinatory voice. Put differently, the more the narrator appears to operate autonomously, the more the observer becomes aware of it as an alien presence. What is especially interesting in Lori Schiller's case is that the mostly indifferent narrator, which mostly comments neutrally on her experience, sometimes becomes very critical, even ominous, threatening, and harassing. What makes the narrator's voice so alien is that its volume gets turned up periodically to the point of creating a distraction, forcing her to pay attention to it. The reason it becomes an inimicable presence rather than a neutral commentator is that it tells her what she isn't inclined to hear and she can't turn the volume down or the sound off. The narrator continues to do what it always does, commenting on her experience, but what she perceives as taunting remarks are merely the narrator giving voice to her feeling of awfulness while she is mentally falling apart. If the narration was a whisper or under her executive control, as it usually is under normal conditions, it would not be viewed as foreign to the self-system. The narrator function keeps trying to preserve some semblance of mental order by weaving an ongoing story about what she is experiencing, but under the spotlight of her attention, it assumes some of the attributes of the other persecuting voices, which represent hallucinations because her self-system doesn't assume ownership of them.

Because of its capacity to deconstruct the self-system, schizophrenia is very instructive for our purposes. With this disorder, all types of strange and disturbing things happen to people. They see imaginary people and hear imaginary voices. Malignant influences are at work to control their thoughts and behaviors or harm them in some undefinable way. They see significance everywhere—in the raised eyebrows of people, in a newspaper headline, in a laugh—and all this somehow applies to them. The world in which they live becomes disturbing and threatening. Inner and outer reality become intertwined, and they lose the capacity to distinguish between them. As one psychotic person aptly put it, "I was so inside myself that everything else, everything outside me, was blurred and unreal."[6]

What makes psychotic experiences so compelling has to do with the heightened sense of meaning that emerges during mental aberrations. This heightened sense of meaning imparts certainty to the perceptions and thoughts of the mentally disturbed and convinces them that what they experience is true and real. This sense of conviction is essential for optimal functioning under such mentally disruptive conditions. If it was lacking, mentally ill persons would be completely incapacitated by their inner mental chaos since they wouldn't know which of their confusing experiences to act on.

In *The Idiot*, Dostoevsky brilliantly describes how this sense of meaning can imbue a clearly aberrant experience in Prince Myshkin with the imprimatur of truth. In the moments before Myshkin has a seizure, his brain seems to catch fire, dispelling his darkness and depression, and flooding his mind and heart with a dazzling light. All his anxieties are transformed into a harmonious joy. Reflecting on these wondrous experiences after his epileptic fit, Myshkin is troubled by the paradox that they were caused by a disease. But then he reasons that is irrelevant. The beauty and perfection he experienced at those precious moments reflected for him an intense heightening of awareness, "the highest synthesis of life," and were worth the whole of his life.[7] As in the case of hallucinatory drugs and schizophrenia, we again find the primal sense of self associated with a compelling, increased awareness, which in turn becomes equivalent with the sense of "I."

THE SENSE OF "ME"

The sense of "me" is that aspect of the self-system that the "I" observes and assumes ownership of. Possessing its own developmental history, it varies from inception to childhood, through adulthood and old age, and represents an accumulation of experiences. It includes all of our changing thoughts, feelings, attitudes, values and behaviors, and sometimes our prized possessions or creative expressions, all those aspects of ourselves that we identify as "mine." It also includes all the imagoes of the important people and role models in our lives that we have incorporated within us. Since many of the workings of our bodies and our minds are usually inaccessible to consciousness, much of the "me" remains unknown to the "I." The part we are most aware of underlies our sense of identity, which not only includes the notion of who we are but also of who we hope to be. The part that others are aware of constitutes our personality, which represents the social vehicle through which we negotiate our needs.

Usually the "I" and the "me," the two main subcomponents within the self-system, operate in synchrony. Under abnormal conditions, though, the "I" and the "me" become partly unlinked and seem to be operating independently as the stream of awareness runs in parallel with the stream of experiences. When this happens, aspects of the "me," such as certain thoughts, feelings, or perceptions, may be experienced as alien presences of the "not-me."

This tendency to regard parts of our own experiences as foreign is common in obsessive-compulsive disorders. Take the case of a woman I knew, a member of a fundamentalist church, who became progressively distraught and incapacitated by her obsessive thoughts. Whenever she saw a word, she felt obliged to spell it and then compare it to other words, trying to decide which was better. This made driving difficult, because when she saw a sign she became distracted. If she saw an ad on television, which said "toll-free," she would pick out "free" because it meant salvation to her. If someone on TV said "rape," she would have to change that in her mind to "tape," because that was a better word. She also claimed to be constantly battling the demons who called her bad names and put thoughts in her mind, like "Why don't you kill yourself?" or "You're no good," or "You committed the unpardonable sin." She believed that her condition was caused by the Devil, who sent all those evil spirits to keep her from working for God, and she spent most of her waking moments mentally beseeching Beelzebub to leave her alone.

In time, these obsessions metastasized to almost all aspects of her mental processes, including her thoughts, images, and decision-making. Mostly, these runaway thoughts had to do with obscene, blasphemous, or other socially taboo themes. Once a train of thought started, it had to be concluded without interruption or else she became irritable and anxious. Each idea or theme had to be counterbalanced by its opposite or some presumed antidote, often paralyzing her with doubts. Because she equated her thoughts with actual deeds, she felt compelled to neutralize them through repetitive, compulsive behavior, such as counting or praying.

Here is another account of certain mental experiences associated with an obsessive thought disorder. The sane voices inside this person's head loudly shouted her every thought "with a rapidity of action that resembled . . . the sudden collapse of a card-house falling down."[8] In contrast, the mad voices never said what she was thinking. They said things contrary to her own thoughts and opinions. They astonished her. "They said things that I never had, and never should have, thought—and all this while I myself was thinking my own, quite independent thoughts."[9]

While some professionals still claim that obsessive- compulsive behavior of this sort can be produced by psychological conflicts, some of the advances in modern psychopharmacology suggest a deficiency of the brain neurotransmitter serotonin as a potential cause. Evidence for an underlying physical basis for these symptoms is strong. Obsessions and compulsions are commonly found in persons with Tourette's syndrome, a neurological disorder characterized by assorted bodily and facial tics as well as uncontrolled grunts, sounds, and often obscene verbal ejaculations. Obsessive ruminations are prominent as an aftermath of encephalitis lethargica, commonly known as sleeping sickness. Thoughts, which have certain characteristics of obsessions, also can be produced through electrical stimulation of the brain. When a neurosurgeon, for example, stimulates an electrode placed in the brain of a conscious patient and causes his hand to move or makes him vocalize or have a memory, the patient identifies the surgeon and not himself as the perpetrator of the experience. The experience is his, yet it is not. He only adopts it as his own when he perceives his "I" as his own internal stimulator.

What, then, do the mental disruptions caused by obsessions and compulsions tell us about the operation of the self-system, and particularly the sense of "me"?

First, people who suffer from this condition have almost an incapacitating hyperawareness of their own perceptions, thought processes, and behaviors, resulting in a deautomatization and fragmentation of behavior, much as might happen if a pianist tried to play a concerto while thinking about how each of his fingers worked. What distinguishes these conditions from psychoses, such as schizophrenia, is that the self-reflective function of the self remains intact since sufferers are usually aware that their obsessions and compulsions are irrational, even though they feel compelled to act on them. In a sense, they become helpless spectators and merciless critics of their own experiences.

Second, we find that perceptions, thoughts, fantasies, and behaviors seemingly can operate independently of one another and, most important, of the internal governor within the self-system. At the same time, these mental processes are capable of operating simultaneously on two or more separate tracks. On one track, people can pursue one train of thought, while on another track, they can be arguing constantly with what they think, while on yet another track, they may be disgusted with themselves for engaging in this futile and irrational discourse. What this suggests is that while the thought processes we identify as part of our "me" operate most smoothly and effectively when no competing ones exist, it's possible for other sometimes contradictory programs to run simultaneously in our minds. When that happens, the "I" works at establishing which train of thought is its own and which is alien, even though each may reflect a different aspect of the self.

Third, when people have thoughts, feelings, or fantasies that run counter to their basic values, they automatically try to counter or neutralize them in much the same manner antibodies respond to germs. Doing battle with foreign invaders is the natural response of the self-system at every level, bodily and psychologically, even if what is identified as foreign really is not. Misidentifications of this sort, as we noted before, occur in various autoimmune diseases, such as lupus, rheumatoid arthritis, or multiple sclerosis.

What all this adds up to is that for the smoothest operation of the self-system, the "I" and the "me" subsystems need to function in unison as the "I-me." When this happens, the beam of awareness cast by the observer function of the "I" on the experiences of the "me" becomes dim and the mental commentary by the internal narrator is in whispers. This is characteristic of normal mental functioning. When the "I-me" become disengaged due to a disruption in this self-system, the whispers turn to shouts as the beam of awareness focuses more intensely on certain experiences of the "me" and treats them as foreign intruders.

Other mental disorders give us further important insights about the operation of the self-system. Dissociative disorders, for example, reveal that different "me's" can exist within the self-system. The sense of "I" need not be confined to experiences of a particular "me" that are associated with a particular personal identity. As we noted before, awareness, which is integral to the observer functions of the "I," has no personal history or identity. Therefore, the same sense of "I" can be transferred to different "me's" within the self-system, even though certain of the "me's" may not be accessible to knowledge by others.

Unlike obsessional states, in which people are hyperaware of their mental processes, dissociative states are characterized by a selective hypoawareness. When certain sets of experience are illuminated by the beam of awareness, other sets are kept in the dark. The compartmentalizing of different parts of the mind—thoughts, feelings and intentions—results in the quasi-independent, autonomous operation of each, often without any conscious awareness. This often can involve complex behaviors, such as happens during trances or highway hypnosis, when we lose all memory of driving over long stretches of road.

With dissociative states, such as multiple personality, there is no warring between the "I" and the "me" as there is in obsessional conditions. No conflicts exist within the "I" subsystem, which assumes ownership for the particular thoughts, feelings, and perceptions within each of the different compartments of the "me." All activities of the "me," even though separated, fall within the bailiwick of the "I." It is the "me" subsystem that becomes unstable, crystallizing into partly overlapping but separate psychological entities that resist full integration with the others, even though they inhabit the same brain.

Because the sense of "I" can align itself with different constellations of experiences within the "me" subsystem without working to reconcile any contradictions among them, it's no surprise that dissociative states accommodate themselves so well to visitations by outside agencies, such as guiding spirits or demons, or underlie out-of-body experiences, such as during shamanistic trances or profound meditative states. With the suspension of critical faculties and the absence of an inner overseer, dissociative states often leave a mental vacuum of power, inviting charismatic leaders or preachers to assume control by offering their own narrations as substitutes for those of the people who are entranced. The amnesia which is such a prominent feature of dissociation suggests that we retain a sense of self only for those experiences illuminated by awareness or accessible to our memory.

"You point out that for Virginia Woolf a great part of every day is not lived consciously, 'that non-being alternates with separate moments of being and that her connection, periods of connection with the world, alternate with fugue-like states,'" I commented to Louise DeSalvo. "Now from my perception, this seems like somebody who is not coping adequately and who is flitting in and out of dissociative states when dealing with unpleasant reality and her problems. How do you mesh those observations with your view that she's coping well?"

"It's extremely complicated, because Virginia Woolf is an incest survivor," DeSalvo responded. "To say that a survivor is not coping adequately is to me to misunderstand the normal, because the sequelae to acts of violence are fugue-like states. Now I take it a step from there. In the face of this act, virtually all incest survivors develop these patterns. The issue is, what is the person doing about that? Is the person struggling to understand her responses? Is the person actively trying to cope, given the fact that a sense of futility is also a common outgrowth of the incest experience? My feeling is that you need to understand the courage this woman showed in trying to understand what this situation was about. . . . So I see these states as adaptive. The only problem is that there are tremendous consequences to the psyche for using this kind of adaptation. I think she struggled to understand it."

The mood disorders illustrate other characteristics of the sense of "me." Along with their euphoria and grandiosity, manics tend to think at a pace that often gets far ahead of themselves. Spilling over with plans, ideas, and schemes, they seek out other people to share them. They often can't stand to be alone. They need people to talk to, to seduce, or to admire them. Sometimes, in its more severe forms, when accompanied by poor judgment and excesses, mania leaves in its wake a confused, embarrassed, and shaken person with painful doubts about herself. "Which of my feelings is real?" Kay R. Jamison, a noted psychologist, would wonder after one of her serious bouts. "Which of the me's is me?"[10] In milder forms of mania, this unbounded sense of self often seems well-suited to poetic expression. With their senses so alive and the world so pregnant with meaning, individuals often can hardly contain themselves. The boundaries of their self-system seem to be bursting at the seams. A woman poet I know described these feelings well.

> I can't put the lid on.
>
> The drawer is too stuffed.
> The closet is jammed.
>
> The weeds are too high.
> The flowers are too many.
>
> The hat is too small.
> The suit is too tailored.
>
> The bubbles now bubble.
> The wine popped its cork.
>
> The tub overflowed.
> The roof sprung a leak.
>
> The pot boiled over.
> And I still can't put the lid on!
>
> I no longer fit myself!!

Depression, in contrast, seems to slow down all aspects of the self-system, except for the ongoing, morbid thoughts, which become accentuated by the inner narrator. The stream of thought becomes sluggish, motivation diminishes, and social interaction decreases. The boundaries of the self retract as the black hole of depression causes the self to collapse upon itself. People feel worthless, deficient, and flawed. The monitoring and executive functions of the self-system stand by ineffectually as morbid thoughts and the anguish of melancholia take on a life of their own. Nothing seems to matter. Living becomes painful, sometimes almost too much to endure.

While the "I" subsystem understandably seems to identify milder forms of mania as compatible or familiar, probably because it induces moods and behaviors that are consonant with our underlying desires to feel good and be productive, it tends to regard depression as unwanted and foreign. When depression occurs, along with its morbid thoughts and physical changes, it becomes an alien part of the "me" subsystem because it doesn't match our inner expectations about how we're supposed to feel, unless of course, we've been depressed for most of our lives or have good reasons to be depressed. Winston Churchill, for instance, referred to his bouts of melancholia as attacks by the "black dog." Tracy Thompson, a staff reporter for *The Washington Post* who viewed her depression (which she called "the Beast") as symptomatic of a defective brain, wondered what distinguished her sense of "I" from the brain it owned. "Maybe it was that healthy part of my brain," she concluded, "which kept trying to say, 'There is something wrong here'—but kept getting misunderstood and tangled in its own messages.'"[11]

The radical act of suicide, most often associated with depression, reveals another dimension of the self-system: the powerful tendency of the "I" subsystem to retain awareness and perpetuate itself despite the painful experiences associated with the "me." Given the property of all living systems to resist extinction, the question is, who kills whom when people take their own lives? Does the self-system in its entirety seek its own self-destruction? Or does some component of it act to destroy the remainder? If life is truly meaningless for people, then suicide should not be a viable option. Inactivity or immobilization should be the natural response to meaninglessness. The very decision of people to kill themselves paradoxically argues against the lack of meaning.[12] As we observed before, suicide means that the person has decided that "life isn't worth it" or "the pain of living is too great" or "I don't deserve to live" or "my family will be better off without me"—all conclusions loaded with meaning. Because of this apparent contradiction within the self-system, a self-preservative function remains at work, continuously finding reasons for living despite the suicidal preoccupations of people, sometimes insuring that their attempts at suicide will be flawed or that they will be prevented from taking their lives by inducing them to issue disguised calls for help or arranging for them to try killing themselves when successful intervention is likely. Of course, when the inner pain becomes so unbearable and intractable in these individuals, the prospects of oblivion and relief may drown out their biological imperative for life.

In an account of his depression, William Styron gave a vivid description of the monitoring component of his self-system—"a wraithlike observer who, not sharing the dementia of his double, is able to watch with dispassionate curiosity as his companion struggles against the oncoming disaster, or decides to embrace it. There is a theatrical quality about all this, and during the next several days, as I went about stolidly preparing for extinction, I couldn't shake off a sense of melodrama—a melodrama in which I, the victim-to-be of self-murder, was both the solitary actor and lone member of the audience. I had not yet chosen the mode of my departure, but I knew that that step would come next, and soon, as inescapable as nightfall."[13]

That the executive function at the helm of the self-system can act to keep the entire organizational structure afloat despite the mutiny of its crew is shown by the many instances of failed suicide. In her ill-disguised autobiography, *The Bell Jar*, Sylvia Plath described this self-preservative action in operation during two failed suicide attempts. On the first occasion she tried to hang herself. She took the silk cord of her mother's yellow bathrobe, fashioned it into a slipknot, and hunted for a place to attach the rope in the low-ceilinged house. After a discouraging time of walking about with the silk cord dangling from her neck like a yellow cat's tail and finding no place to fasten it, she sat on the edge of her mother's bed and tried pulling the cord tight.

"But each time I would get the cord so tight I could feel a rushing in my ears and a flush of blood in my face, my hands would weaken and let go, and I would be all right again.

"Then I saw that my body had all sorts of little tricks, such as making my hands go limp at the crucial second, which would save it, time and again, whereas if I had the whole say, I would be dead in a flash.

"I would simply have to ambush it with whatever sense I had left, or it would trap me in its stupid cage for fifty years without any sense at all. And when people found out my mind had gone, as they would have to sooner or later, in spite of my mother's guarded tongue, they would persuade her to put me into an asylum where I could be cured.

"Only my case was incurable."[14]

On another occasion, she decided to drown herself while she was swimming in the sea. She brought her hands to her breast, ducked her head, and dived, using her hands to push the water aside. The water pressed in on her eardrums and on her heart. She fanned herself down, but before she knew where she was the water had spat her up into the sun, and the world was sparkling all about her like blue and green and yellow semi-precious stones.

"I dashed the water from my eyes," the heroine proclaimed.

"I was panting, as after a strenuous exertion, but floating, without effort.

"I dived, and dived again, and each time popped up like a cork.

"The grey rock mocked me, bobbing on the water easy as a life buoy.

"I knew when I was beaten.

"I turned back."[15]

As it happened, Sylvia Plath eventually did manage to take her life years later by sticking her head in an oven after swallowing a quantity of sleeping pills, but she did so after days if not weeks of sending off many ill-disguised messages of her intentions, seemingly inviting someone to intervene. Three days before her suicide, she was seen several times by her psychiatrist, who was alarmed enough about her to want to hospitalize her. Unfortunately, no beds were available, so he made special arrangements to see her as an outpatient on Saturday and Sunday. On Sunday evening, she went to a nearby professor's flat on the pretext of buying postage stamps from him. Ten minutes after she left, the professor opened his door and found her still standing in the hall, as if in a trance. He was enough concerned about her behavior to want to call a doctor. She declined, according to Linda Wagner-Martin, her biographer, and said she was having a wonderful dream, a marvelous vision.[16] What the vision was, she never did say, but it apparently was inviting enough shortly afterwards to induce her to extinguish her creative light forever and leave her beloved children behind.

The struggles of William Styron and Sylvia Plath are instructive. They reveal the tendency in depression for the "I" subsystem within the self to disassociate itself from the morbid thoughts and feelings within the "me," while at the same time acting to preserve itself. Since emotional anguish is so self-absorbing, the "I" subsystem simply seems to be trying to rid itself of a powerful distraction that keeps it from optimally doing its work. These competing forces within the self-system—the tendency to seek relief from pain emanating from the "me" and the urge for self-preservation, which is a property of life itself—apparently accounts for the failed attempts at suicide. The "I" subsystem doesn't seek to extinguish consciousness, one of its main properties. To do so would be as preposterous as the heart working to stop its own beat. When the emotional anguish gets too great, the sense of "I," along with its monitoring and preservative functions, becomes swallowed up by the pain, and the act of self-destruction becomes equivalent to relief.

THE SENSE OF "I-BUT-NOT-ME"

The sense of "I" can be better grasped if we contrast it against its opposite: white against black, heat against cold, good against evil, matter against anti-matter, and as it happens, the self against the non-self. What makes our existence so precious is the immanent prospect of our nonexistence. The reason we are keenly aware of our consciousness is that nightly the reticular activating mechanism within our brainstems turns the illumination off as we unconsciously "experience" nonexperience. Not surprisingly, then, our sense of "I" becomes most expansive when it is not fettered by its linkage with the experiences of our "me." This ability for our awareness to cast aside the anchors of our bodily and mental experiences underlies the spiritual aspects of our selves. Our inclination to believe in a cosmic consciousness or universal being may stem from our desire to counter death, but under certain circumstances, the operation of our self-system lends credence to this inclination. This is especially so during brain disturbances or madness.[17] Commonly, during acute mania or schizophrenia or during the agony of despair, individuals are apt to assign religious significance to their experiences. God speaks personally to them, they have visions of Jesus or the Mother Mary, they acquire supernatural powers, or they believe they have a divine mission. The paradox is not that those who suffer emotionally should turn to God for relief but that some of those who are mentally ill should believe they themselves are God, possess His power, or are His special messengers.

Here is an excerpt from the diary of Vaslav Nijinsky, the famous dancer who suffered from schizophrenia. "The world was made by God. Man was made by God. I am both God and man. I am God, I am God, I am God. . . ."[18] Later, he wrote, "I feel what Christ felt. I am like Buddha, I am the Buddhist God and every kind of God. I know each of them. I pretend to be mad for my own purposes. I am a madman who loves mankind. *My madness is my love towards mankind.*"[19]

John Custance, a writer who suffered from manic-depressive disorder, felt himself so close to God during mania that he wrote, "I am God. I see the future, plan the Universe, save mankind; I am utterly and completely unmortal; I am even male and female. The whole Universe, animate and inanimate, is within me."[20] Later, when sane, he recognized his delusions of grandeur, confessing that, in retrospect, his sense of identity with God seemed to be an appalling blasphemy.

Dissociative states appear ideally suited for the countless religious healings and conversion experiences reported at evangelical and revival services. With no unifying sense of "I" that bridges all waking mental states of the "me," dissociative trances invite the intervention of some external "I," perhaps a charismatic religious leader, who induces entranced members of the congregation to experience the Holy Spirit.

Despair and helplessness are also conducive to religious experiences. Supposedly, 10 percent of all AA recoveries happen through a "rapid awakening," usually of a religious nature. From my research on this topic, this is more likely to occur when the person "hits bottom" or is in the throes of despair. "Man's extremity is God's opportunity," so the saying goes. The former Senator Harold E. Hughes, for example, gave a dramatic account of a religious experience that took place during his battle with alcoholism. Filled with a horrible self-loathing, he picked up his twelve-gauge, single-barrel Remington pump gun one evening, slid three shells in the magazine, pumped one into the chamber, and climbed into his old-fashioned, claw-footed tub. With the shotgun resting on his stomach, he positioned the muzzle in his mouth toward his brain and placed his thumb on the trigger. A terrible sadness filled him. "Oh, God," he groaned, "I'm a failure, a drunk, a liar, and a cheat. I'm lost and hopeless and want to die. Forgive me for doing this." Then he began sobbing convulsively. Once he became exhausted, a strange peace settled deep within him, filling the emptiness. God was reaching down and touching him, a God who cared, a God who loved him.

An intense joy welled up within him. Slowly he rose to his knees and cried out in gratitude, "Whatever You ask me to do, Father, I will do it."[21]

There is no way to know whether God did or did not talk with the former Senator Hughes, but there is another possibility that we also need to consider. As in other instances of severe depression, when the potential for suicide threatens, we have seen the various life-sustaining strategies of the "I" subsystem, which probably derive from biological and cultural programming, automatically kick in to preserve the self. Possibly, when someone feels so miserable and impotent, the commanding or inspiring hallucinatory voice he hears is simply the self-preserving part of the "I," ingeniously intervening as God might do if He cared and telling him exactly what he wanted to hear. Now he doesn't have to kill himself. And with God taking a personal interest in him, he will be able to stop drinking.

It isn't my intention to distinguish "authentic" religious experiences from delusions but simply to examine why this relationship exists and what it says about the nature of the self. As it happens, the common denominator in all these experiences is an alteration in consciousness. With emotional upheavals, drug intoxications, acute psychoses, or serious disturbances in brain function due to alcohol withdrawal, dislocations in the self-system occur, with the sense of "I" becoming disengaged from the sense of "me." This disruption is something that many mystics deliberately try to achieve through drastic means, such as denying their flesh, asceticism, starvation, isolation, and various meditation techniques. When this disruption in bodily boundaries happens, the sense of "I" leaves its corporeal and mental constraints and expands to fill the universal void. They may experience eternity, but always with a glimmer of themselves, not someone else. If they don't identify the experience as their own, it won't hold any value for them when their sense of "I" eventually returns to reclaim the experiences associated with their sense of "me."

These transcendental or mystical experiences, which are usually accompanied by a feeling of rapture or "eureka," have a powerful effect on people. They serve as validations of their spiritual nature. By giving up their identities—those attributes associated with their sense of "me"—they can become part of something much greater than themselves and still retain an awareness about what is transpiring. Paradoxically, the more selfless they become, the more eternal, omniscient, and god-like they're apt to feel. Psychotic, intoxicated, or delirious people, or those who deliberately use techniques to disturb their brain functioning, seem most disposed to divine experiences. This is perhaps why the ancients often regarded madness as a means to supernatural knowledge.

REASSEMBLING THE PARTS

After examining how the self-system operates when any of its important elements is missing or doesn't work, we are in a better position to understand the nature of the self. What these various natural experiments with madness or brain disturbances reveal is that the self, which ordinarily functions as a cohesive and integrated system, has two main subsystems, one comprising the sense of "I" and the other comprising the sense of "me," each with different components. The components that comprise the "I" subsystem are largely responsible for shaping and giving meaning to various activities of the self. They do this through their monitoring, narrating, and governing functions, which process input from the "me." The components that comprise the "me" subsystem include all of the conscious and unconscious activities of the body and mind that contribute to the sense of identity. Unlike the various functions of the "me," which have temporal courses and developmental histories, preceding from the past to the present and future, the beam of awareness of the "I," except for diurnal fluctuations in depth, the dulling effects of fatigue, and the temporary unawareness of sleep, simply remains on continuously unless affected by brain disease or death.

Because the electrocortical activity of the language and speech centers within the brain—Wernicke's area within the temporal lobe and Broca's area within the prefrontal gyrus—is continuous and parallels activity in other areas, the narrator function within the "I" subsystem seems inextricably linked to all those activities of the "me" subsystem that are capable of awareness or being experienced. Acting much like a biographer, the "I" offers an ongoing narrative structure to our various experiences as a way of imbuing them with a sense of continuity, causality, and meaning as it moves our personal life story along. Though these ongoing narrative activities are mostly subvocal and silent and occur at a low level of awareness, they can become highlighted when the observing component of the "I" shifts its beam to them. The chronicling function of the "I" doesn't operate in an executive fashion, like a homunculus, creating stories, manufacturing plans, or setting goals for us. Rather, it tells our story extemporaneously as it is unfolding and makes adjustments in accord with the various plans and programs that shape our activities, experiences, and actions.

Immediately, some will argue that there is no need to propose the existence of a narrator function separate from the thought processes themselves. Ordinarily, with an intact self-system, the narrator function interacts silently and smoothly, with all the activities of the "me" subsystem and distinctions between the "I" and the "me" subsystems superfluous. Under normal conditions, this ongoing commentary about mental activities is unobtrusive, silently chronicling and shaping all conscious mental activity to preserve the story flow before transcribing it into memory. But as certain forms of psychopathology reveal, the narrator function can be teased apart from the thought processes, simultaneously commenting on the flow of thought, sometimes with hallucinatory vividness and the voice of a harsh critic.

Another component of the "I" involves the observer function that, under normal conditions, operates in conjunction with the ongoing biographical activities of the narrator. This spectator function is mostly dispassionate and non-judgmental, simply illumining different aspects of the self-system that require awareness at the moment. With certain kinds of psychopathology, though, the various components within the "I" can become unlinked, and the observer function not only casts its beam of awareness over all functions associated with the "me"—perceptual processes, subjective experiences, and physical activities—but even the operations of the narrator function itself. With profound alterations in consciousness caused by hallucinogens, delirium, meditation, or trance, it can exist as almost pure awareness or illumination, disconnected from any of the activities associated with the self-system. This sense of pure awareness seems to underlie the states of Nirvana, samadhi, or cosmic consciousness sought after by the mystics. At a more mundane level, the observer and narrator functions may work in concert to heighten self-consciousness when they become critical spectators during social interactions or, even more inhibiting, during the sexual act.

Under normal conditions, the components of the "me" operate automatically and in concert. However, with different kinds of mental pathology, the inbuilt regulatory mechanisms within the "me" break down, allowing the different components to operate quasi-independently and out of synch. Thought processes may speed up beyond the ability of the self-system to process them or slow down to a degree that prevents their implementation, or become so fragmented that they interfere with the interpretation of perceptions. Perceptions may become so flooded with meaning as to impede thoughts and actions. People's actions at times may appear to operate independently of their conscious intentions, and they may display various tics, compulsions, or amnesia. People even can engage in complex, seemingly purposeful activities during transient global amnesias, alcoholic blackouts, or complex partial seizures without any awareness or recollection of having done so.

These pathological mental conditions also reveal that the "me" subsystem has the capacity to allow seemingly independent constellations of experience to operate concurrently, much like multitasking in a computer. Under normal conditions, we have the capacity, sometimes referred to as "double think," to entertain incompatible sets of values and beliefs simultaneously without any need to reconcile them logically. If we could not do so, we likely would be at constant war with ourselves since, in the process of growing up, we adopt many attitudes and attributes that are contradictory. This capacity to compartmentalize parts of our minds also happens during dissociative states, which allow the coexistence of seemingly different me's, each with its own set of experiences and behaviors.

"Why did Virginia Woolf use 'Miss Jan' in her diary? Who was she?" I asked Louise DeSalvo.

"I think that very often young writers need to create fictional personae through which to explore issues that relate to themselves. Fiction writers do it all the time. What you try to do is create a fictional persona who will take on some of the issues that you are wrestling with. But because you create a fictional persona, you create a kind of essential distance between yourself and the issues with which you are grappling so that you can begin to look at these issues objectively. I see writing in a diary, for example, as creating the same kind of fictional persona through the same kind of distancing. When we write in a diary, even though it's a personal diary, we create a kind of false persona . . . and I don't mean that in the negative sense. We create a persona who is somewhat different from the self that we are. We create a reflective persona. I see the creation of Ms. Jan in that way, as the creation of a fictional alter ego so that she can begin to examine troubling issues in her life—a sense of who she is in relationship to her family, a sense of why she is suffering so much from the death of a mother, the death of a half-sister. [This was a way for her to grapple] with issues that were incredibly taboo to discuss in the Victorian family."

SELF-REFLECTION

No notion of the self can be adequate unless it accounts for one of the most puzzling abilities of the self: namely, its capacity to reflect upon its own inner workings. While remarkable, this capacity isn't unique, as it first seems, especially if we grant ourselves some leeway in interpretation. When we do, we find that the self-reflective capacity of the self only represents at a psychological level what transpires in all self-regulating biological systems: namely, the capacity to make adjustments on the basis of feedback. For example, though the master pituitary gland (which itself is under the control of the hypothalamus) may control the secretions of the thyroid gland, adrenal glands, parathyroid glands, ovaries, and testes, the hormonal secretions of these glands in turn prompt the pituitary gland to increase or decrease the output of its own regulatory hormones to preserve the homeostatic equilibrium of the entire endocrine system. To preserve homeostasis, excessive activity by one component of the system must prompt corrective feedback by another component of the system. Negative feedback loops of this sort are essential for homeostasis. They also alter our conventional notions of what is meant by executive control. The pituitary gland may be the master gland, but it continually operates under the constraints imposed by the glands it regulates, to preserve the homeostasis of the entire system.

When we extend this self-regulatory property of all biological systems to the self-system, we likewise find that the narrative function of the self operates under similar corrective constraints, imposed by other components of the system, to preserve the homeostasis of the entire self-system during our ongoing activities. No inner homunculus, pygmy executive, or mediating ego exists within the mind, pulling the reins of lesser mental entities. The homeostatic requirements of the system itself regulate the activities of its various components, some of which seem more vital than others. Functioning as a psychological gyroscope, these homeostatic forces automatically make minor adjustments, based on corrective feedback, to maintain equilibrium within the self-system when some part begins to malfunction.

Developments in the field of artificial intelligence offer alternative ways to understand the capacity for self-reflection. With a cybernetic model of intelligence,[22] as well as most neural network or parallel distributed process models, the notion of a recursive loop—a procedure that can repeat itself indefinitely until a specified condition is met—represents the fundamental feedback mechanism within the nervous system.[23] At its simplest level, the feedback loop functions as a reflex arc. As part of a feedback cycle, incoming information is tested against some internal schema, which lets the person identify the stimuli, cluster them into manageable units, fill in missing information, and select a strategy for getting more information to solve a problem or reach a goal.[24] Schemas are prior organizations of learned or genetically programmed knowledge, values, assumptions, or expectations that predispose people to think, feel, and act in certain ways. In parallel distributed processing models of the mind, schemas are not fixed structures. They are flexible configurations, mirroring the regularities of experience, automatically generalizing from the past, and providing automatic completion of missing components, but also adapting continually to reflect the current state of affairs.[25] If an incongruity exists between the incoming information and these internal schemas, the feedback loop keeps operating and retesting the updated information until this difference becomes resolved. With a neural network or parallel distributed processing model of the mind, the self-system becomes adaptive, continually trying to configure itself to match incoming information. The better the match, the more stable the self-system. Activity designed to produce congruence between the available information and the internal schema resembles intentional behavior. Once the incoming information matches the template of the internal schema (or the self-system arrives at a preferred state of interpretation), the testing stops and the particular activity momentarily ceases until more discordant information comes along.

With most biological systems, the match between the incoming information and the inner schema needn't be perfect for the activity to go to completion. There is a good deal of slack in these operations. Though capable of modification, schemas tend to persevere, despite conflicting evidence.[26] Like metaphors, they needn't be perfect to capture the essence of the event. The function of the internal schema is to promote efficiency and not necessarily accuracy in thought and behavior. It is more efficient for us to operate according to general guidelines or road maps than to modify our basic values and assumptive system to conform to each individual exception. Biases, prototypes, and stereotypes allow quicker information processing and behavioral responses. Naturally, when the discrepancy between the incoming information and our inner schema is too large, the self-system becomes highly unstable. Under certain conditions, such as a religious conversion, a serious illness, or a major psychological shock, radical changes in the basic schema may occur.

The matching of incoming information against our inner schema is mostly designed to preserve psychological stability.[27] For us to exist in a changing world and anticipate the future, we require inner plans. Not all plans are conscious or explicit. Unknown biological drives, cultural expectations, and psychological conflicts often influence the course of our actions. Mostly, our plans are vague and sketchy and allow us leeway to maneuver and fill in details. One of the important functions of the self-system is to integrate these various plans into a unified course of action. When certain of these plans are mutually incompatible, such as when personal desires conflict with social expectations, then the self-system is likely to operate less efficiently as it tries to reconcile these differences into a more cohesive plan. When the routine efforts of the self-system to match our perceptions and behavioral outputs against its inner schema and implicit plans aren't successful, it generates thoughts in us that we experience as conscious intentions. What we interpret to be a deliberate course of action on our part, therefore, may simply be automatic problem-solving efforts to restore harmony among the conflicts and incompatibilities within our self-system.

What this means for the self-system is that adjustments and fine-tunings are occurring continuously to align our experiences and plans with the way they are predisposed to be. Ordinarily, we have no conscious awareness of the operation of our selves when this feedback system operates seamlessly, without encountering major incongruities between our ongoing experiences and the inner schema, dispositions, and implicit plans they are matched against. At these times, we seem to be operating spontaneously and feel "at one with ourselves." Only when our thoughts, feelings, and actions are substantially discrepant with our internal schema or plans do we become acutely self-conscious and feel compelled to restore inner equilibrium. When the self-system shifts from automatic pilot to more purposive control of the activities of the "me" in order to reduce conflict, the sense of "I" becomes heightened. Paradoxically, then, we're likely to feel most at one with ourselves when we're least aware of our own thought processes and most at odds with ourselves when we become unintentional observers of them.

What these so-called "natural experiments" with mental illness also reveal is that the self-system, just as other biological systems, can't always compensate for deficiencies in its component parts. When the regulatory mechanisms fail, homeostasis can't always be maintained. Positive feedback loops may develop and cause the system to break down. Within the endocrine system, for example, pathology in the thyroid gland may cause it to operate independently of pituitary and hypothalamic control. With hypothyroidism or hyperthyroidism, it will continue to secrete abnormally low or abnormally large amounts of thyroid hormones, respectively, despite the compensatory attempts of the pituitary to become more or less active to maintain normal secretory levels. Similarly, within the self-system, positive feedback loops may develop, which amplify rather than dampen deviations from normal homeostasis. Our emotions may take on a life of their own with depression as we become depressed about being depressed, or our thought processes may take on a life of their own with obsessions as we generate thoughts to counter unpleasant thoughts, or our fears may worsen with phobias as we become more anxious about being afraid. The very attempt to resist hallucinatory voices or stop compulsive behaviors may perpetuate and worsen them. When this internal feedback loop malfunctions, the homeostatic forces within the self-system futilely keep spinning potentially suitable solutions, as probably happens in the tortuous and convoluted thought processes of neurotics, in an attempt to resolve discrepancies and move the narrative flow of experience along.

This self-reflexive or self-reflecting attribute of the self has implications far beyond the capacity for maintaining homeostasis of the self-system through corrective feedback. In his imaginative book, *Gödel, Escher, Bach: An Eternal Golden Braid*, Douglas Hofstadter claims that the ability of the self to reflect upon itself argues for a novel notion of causality in which events at one level of organization can be translated automatically into events at another level of organization or simultaneously can lead to other events at the same level.[28] At a biological level of our existence, for instance, a strictly deterministic or probabilistic program may run, which at a higher psychological level we experience as free-will, intuition, or creativity. Hofstadter views this seeming paradox as a form of "strange loop" or "tangled hierarchy." Like an Escher drawing or a Bach fugue that can seamlessly end up where it began, a strange loop phenomenon or tangled hierarchy happens whenever we unexpectedly find ourselves back where we started after moving upwards or backwards through the levels of some hierarchical system. The illusion is created because a level is shielded from our view and offers an element of surprise.

Escher's lithograph *Drawing Hands* illustrates this illusion. As we study the lithograph, we get drawn into the tangled hierarchy of symbols, where thoughts flow back and forth. This is the elusive level of the mind. At this conscious or visible level, we become aware that each hand, like the ability of the self to reflect upon itself, impossibly seems to be creating the other. According to Hofstadter, the strange loop is created by our perception that something in the system emerges from the system and acts on the system as though it was outside the system. What is so ingenious about this drawing is that it momentarily paralyzes our critical faculties because the illusion is at several levels. The first is of the hands coming out of the drawing. They aren't supposed to do that. The second is that each hand holds a pencil, which is an object for creation. If instead each

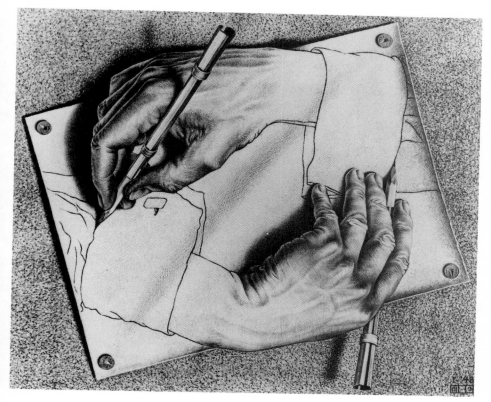

hand held a bar of soap and was washing the other arm, the illusion wouldn't be as startling at the symbolic level. The third is the invisible level, the one easily forgotten in any analysis of the drawing. This has to do with the existence of the artist who draws the hands drawing each other. At this invisible level, no illusion or mystery exists. The artist simply constructs a drawing in the same manner that other artists do, only the nature of the drawing causes us to overlook that. However, if we wish to add even more complexity to Hofstadter's analysis, we can ask what inner function inspired Escher to create the drawing hands creating each other, but that brings us into the logical absurdity of infinite regress.

What the analysis of this drawing reveals so well is the different levels at which our minds operate. Our thoughts may operate entirely on one plane of consciousness, creating new thoughts and proposing new theories, without awareness of hidden levels of neural activity or biological programming, which unduly bias our perspectives. The seeming impossibility of a self reflecting upon itself may be no more mysterious than this Escher drawing. Only in the case of self-reflection, we have no idea of who or what is responsible for creating the illusion.

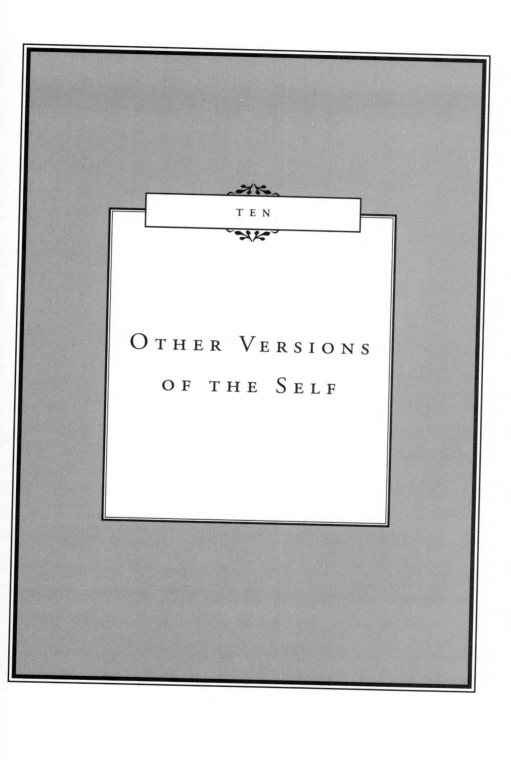

TEN

OTHER VERSIONS

OF THE SELF

SURELY, IN YOUR MUSINGS, you've wondered about the difference in your life if you had made one fateful decision rather than another. Would you now be a different person or more or less happy if you married X instead of Y, if you pursued this career instead of that, if you opted to have or not to have children, if you made this move rather than that, or if you acted or hadn't acted on your convictions? Without reliving your life, you never can be sure, but you can get an inkling of what the differences might have been by using your imagination.

Take the case of Rebecca. As a child, she was active and bright and curious and eager to please and easily hurt. She excelled in school and engaged in many extracurricular activities but never felt pretty or popular or smart enough to be secure. Though she loved both of her parents, she felt intimidated by her father, a successful, outspoken businessman, and emotionally drawn toward her mother, an intelligent and unhappy housewife whose role attracted and repelled her. Vaguely discontented, she looked toward college as her entrance into adulthood, an avenue to pursue her interests in literature and perhaps meet someone nice there. She found college life exciting, especially being on her own, but in her junior year she faced a difficult dilemma. She had been dating two boys, but felt pressed to make a choice between them.

Scott was a law student, confident and ambitious, someone who could provide her with the style of life she was used to. She liked him very much, even though he was against her pursuing a career in journalism. He eventually wanted to set up practice in his home town and start a family and didn't think his wife should work.

Then there was Mark, exceptionally talented in art and fiercely independent. The times they spent together were exciting and fun and sometimes upsetting and filled with intense and often heated intellectual debates. But imagining a future life with him was scary because of the economic uncertainties and his insistence on an unconventional life without children.

Let's briefly play out two different scenarios.

Scenario No. 1. Rebecca eventually marries Scott and leads a respectable, middle-class life expected from the wife of an up-and-coming young lawyer: being active in church affairs, doing volunteer work, getting involved in the P.T.A., and entertaining socially. Although she has a nice home, nice children, nice friends, a nice husband, and a nice life, she is unhappy. Over the years, her spells of depression and irritability worsen, and she feels guilty because she has no reason to feel that way. Perhaps, when the children go off to college, she tells herself, she'll find an interesting job, or maybe try to write. Maybe that will help. Maybe.

Scenario No. 2. Rebecca lives with Mark, despite her parents' disapproval, and with his encouragement pursues a master's degree in journalism. Times are financially hard since Mark has trouble selling any paintings and her parents refuse to help out, angry with her because of her unconventional way of life. They both take odd jobs and manage to scrape by, but this doesn't bother her too much since many of their friends are in the same boat. Then one day, after submitting numerous applications and going to countless job interviews, the big break happens for her. A well-known newspaper in New York offers her a job. Ecstatic, Mark and Rebecca decide to celebrate by getting married. The move is no problem for Mark since he can paint anywhere, and besides, New York is where all the action is in the art world. They find a small apartment in Greenwich Village and get settled. In time, both of their careers thrive. Eventually, after writing a successful column and doing some freelance work, Rebecca becomes general editor of an experimental literary journal, and Mark finally gets an excellent gallery to represent him and makes some big sales. Life is exciting and full for Rebecca. This is the fabled life she always dreamed of. Many interesting and creative friends, some of whom are important celebrities. The thrill of living in the center of culture and entertainment, and beginning to earn enough money to enjoy it. A witty and brilliant husband, temperamental and impossible at times, but still her best friend. Yet for all the glitter in her life, she still feels a periodic emptiness and melancholy, a sense of not being fulfilled. Sometimes smoking a joint helps, but mostly it makes her feel worse. She wonders whether the alienation from her parents is part of the problem and wishes the family could be close again—but this seems hopeless, since every time her father and Mark get together they end up arguing. She wonders whether their decision not to have children is at the root of her discontent, but dismisses the thought, realizing there is no way having a child can fit into their lifestyle. Maybe she is working too hard, maybe she needs to take a long vacation, as her husband suggests. Maybe that will help. Maybe.

Now let's merge these two scenarios by imagining that Rebecca No. 1, on a trip to New York with some other ladies in her church, by accident happens to sit next to Rebecca No. 2 during lunch at the cafeteria in the Museum of Modern Art. Prompted by a vague sense of recognition, Rebecca No. 1 turns to her chic and attractive tablemate and engages her in conversation. Rebecca No. 2, experiencing an initial, magnetic pull towards the woman next to her, pleasantly inquires about the other's life. But then, after a brief exchange, one becomes cool and the other bored as they both finish their food in polite, estranged silence.

Here they sit, both alike, but not liking the other. They are both at a similar point in their lives, experience a similar, vague discontent, yet find that they have little in common. And with good reason. Their entire world view seems different. Not only does Rebecca No. 1 center her life on her children and husband, but her small town provincialism and conservatism and church involvement are far different from the cosmopolitanism and liberalism and agnosticism of her biological double. Because each Rebecca now inhabits an entirely different story, each one seemingly contradictory and threatening to the credibility of the other, they don't even make the effort to learn that they share a common heritage, possess a similar need to please others and be liked, have similar temperaments, and rely on the same physical and intellectual endowments to live their lives. Though biologically identical, they now appear to be entirely different people because of the choices each has made.

Of course, the use of one major decision point to illustrate a radical alteration in life course is overly simplistic, since in most instances, countless smaller and less obvious choices are involved. But this still demonstrates an important point. Certain key decisions can lead people to become different versions of themselves.

This anecdote raises important issues about the self. The first has to do with whether someone remains the same person no matter what course he or she pursues in life. Undoubtedly, as the results of studies on identical twins who have been adopted separately at infancy and reared apart reveal, genetics is a powerful predictor of later behavior.[1] But it isn't an absolute determinant. Identical twins don't always turned out to be identical. If they were, then if one developed a genetically linked ailment, such as schizophrenia, then the other one would as well. However, since this happens in less that 50 percent of the cases, environmental forces must modify even outcomes such as mental illness.

So even if the two versions of Rebecca are biological replicas, we needn't expect them to be absolutely identical in temperament or outlook, especially after exposure to different life experiences. The initial attraction and later dislike that transpired between the two versions of Rebecca during their chance meeting at the M.O.M.A. isn't so dissimilar from what can happen between the different identities of a multiple personality, which may be protective of, indifferent to, or antagonistic toward the primary one. This suggests, as Virginia Woolf observed, that people possess a potential multiplicity of selves that can come into being under different circumstances. Some of these selves may display characteristics similar to or at variance with those of other potential selves.

What this anecdote shows, as does the phenomenon of multiple personality, is that while potential versions of the self share many commonalities, some versions may turn out to be incompatible with others. As sometimes happens, they even may develop so much antipathy between them that one wishes to destroy the other. The actual case of the Nicholson twins illustrates this well.[2]

Almost inseparable since birth, Todd and Timothy seemed to have interwoven identities. As young children, when one looked in the mirror he saw the other. Throughout their childhood, they dressed alike and were constant companions, often showing an almost telepathic understanding of each other's needs and thoughts. They were so alike that, as pranks, they often would switch places on dates and in the bedroom. As seemed inevitable, they entered business together as partners and then, as a way of showing some independence, also developed successful enterprises on their own. But under the surface of this seeming harmony and closeness, other interactions took place. The relationship between the brothers was marked by constant friction and tension. There were many instances when one bullied and threatened the other and when they temporarily severed their relationship, only to become reconciled again. The animosity between them became so great that one day Timothy shot and killed his brother. At his trial, he claimed that the shooting was accidental. However, the fact that two bullets were found in the victim and that he once tried to hire someone to kill his brother persuaded the jury otherwise.

What all this means for our two versions of Rebecca is that even with the same biological makeup, temperament, and early life experiences, they turned out later to be two different persons after they entered different personal stories. Extrapolating from this hypothetical situation, we can assume, then, that if we could take widely divergent paths in life, we'd likely turn out to be different versions of ourselves. All of these potential versions would possess the same sense of "I," because they rely on the same brain to generate awareness, store information, and narrate what transpires, but each would have a different sense of "me" because of its accumulated new experiences over time, which should produce distinctive sets of attitudes and values. Also, because of the different people who become important in these various lives, each version's sense of "we" would be affected. Each of these potential selves would have incorporated different people in its particular life story and, as a consequence, would have become enmeshed in their life stories, too.

The point is that there is no such thing as a fixed sense of "me" that remains stable and unchanging throughout our entire lives, independent of the circumstances we encounter, our accumulated experiences, and the choices we make, although it does tend to become more inflexible over time. Early in our lives, when our attitudes and values are being formed and we're learning new ways to process information, the potential is greatest for us to become any one of many different selves. With more and more decisive experiences and more inflexible ways of interpreting them, our options for deviating from our particular course progressively diminish. Except for serious adversity or trauma or major life changes or ill health, which can cause radical shifts and realignments in our attitudes and perceptions, our self-system becomes more and more self-confirming and limits our access to other potential selves.

The extent to which the life experiences and acquired outlook of any of our potential selves are compatible with the basic biological makeup, temperament, and early life programming common to all determines how comfortable that particular version will be with itself. Certain versions will exist harmoniously within certain life stories, while others won't. No single one of these potential versions is any more our "real" self than another. It's simply a different version. We are who we are, but not necessarily all the versions we could have been. The version we happen to be depends on the particular life story we happen to find ourselves in at any particular moment. Only our imagination, which isn't bound by the strictures of causality, lets us go backward and forward in time and wonder about the other versions of ourselves we could have become if only such-and-such happened or we had made such-and-such choice.

I asked David McCullough about the most important shaping influences on Harry Truman.

"There's no question about the two most formative experiences of his life. [One was] when he was recalled by his father, from what seemed like a budding career in banking, to come back to the old farm and work as a farmer, something he had no experience in whatsoever and no particular inclination towards until then. And he spent eleven years working as hard as hell as a farmer, burdened by debt, troubled by all the usual ups and downs of that life—by drought and heat and rain and the wrath of plague and all the rest—and it changed him, no question about it.

"The second great turning point was his experience in the First World War. . . . The Greeks said character is destiny. It might also be said that setting too is destiny."

THE WYSIWYG PRINCIPLE

With any of the potential versions that Rebecca (or we, for that matter) could become, the question is which of them should we regard as the most "authentic"? In the current moral climate, people place a high premium on authenticity. It has become a moral absolute. To be authentic means to be genuine, sincere, and principled, and to act according to our moral convictions. It means being forthright and not having any hidden agendas. It is the WYSIWYG principle in word processing—what you see is what you get—applied to human relations.

Authenticity also is used in another sense. Certain influential writers argue that it represents the truest expression of the self. This most usually comes about through altruism, when we transcend the limits of "self-centered selfhood" or seek "horizons of significance." When we think only for ourselves, as one author put it, we "turn the world into a meaningless desert," but when we think about the welfare of others, we fulfill our true self and give meaning to our existence.[3]

What we find then are contradictory views about what constitutes authenticity. One view sees authenticity as a means of being true to one's self, whatever that self may be. But a second view, which seems quite the opposite, suggests that authenticity means being selfless. In whatever way authenticity is used, it carries a good connotation, something we should strive for, while being inauthentic carries a bad one, the antithesis of the WYSIWYG principle.

Harry S. Truman, a former President of the United States, has been called by many epithets, but even his worst critics were not likely to regard him as devious. Though at times tactless and impolitic, his shoot-from-the-hip style won him many admirers and also made him many enemies. In his way, he was almost an exemplar of what is meant by authentic.

"You made a statement in your book, which I found rather remarkable applied to a politician," I said to David McCullough, Truman's biographer. "You said, 'ambitious by nature, he was never torn by ambition, never tried to appear as something he was not.' Did you really mean that? How could a politician at times not present himself as something he was not?"

"I suppose it's a relative statement compared to the practices of most successful politicians. . . . He did not put on an act. We've just gone through an election where people were trying to act like Harry Truman. If they do that, then they miss the point about him because he never tried to act like anybody else. He never tried to present himself to the public as anyone but Harry Truman. He didn't have any knack for putting on a show, as most successful politicians do.

"And he was also very smart. He was keenly intelligent, and he knew that it wouldn't work, especially so, for example, when he comes on stage after one of the greatest acts of all time, Franklin Roosevelt. F.D.R. was a master at the art of political performance, and he had all the natural endowments. He was handsome. He had a gorgeous voice. He was magnetic and inspirational, all the things Truman wasn't and knew he couldn't be. So that when people tried to coax him to do this or do that, he didn't pay much attention to it.

"Now of course, he wasn't just the same all the time on stage and off stage, because nobody is. He was much more complex than he appeared. . . . All the people I talked to, who knew him both privately and publicly, professionally and intimately, stressed that the man they knew and the man we knew as the President were one and the same. And that *he* knew who he was. That's the most important thing. He said at one point after he had retired back in Independence, "I tried never to forget who I was, where I came from, and where I would go back to." He's grounded, and he likes who he is. . . .

"If you look, for example, at the speeches he made during his Whistle Stop campaign across the country, and particularly the speeches in the small towns, not the big speeches in the big cities, which were prepared in advance, they're nearly all extemporaneous. There are no two the same. He would come out there and just talk to the people in a very straightforward way. In effect he was saying 'Here's what I am, here's what I stand for, make up your own minds.' And it worked, and that's how he won. . . . His seeming genuineness . . . is almost impossible for us to believe today."

Despite its presumed virtues, the notion of authenticity is problematic. From a moral perspective, being selfless or true to our beliefs has no bearing on how others are affected by our actions. Highly principled zealots or fanatics, committed to the greater good as they see it, have perpetrated wars, massacres, inquisitions, crusades, and persecution against others with different religious or political persuasions or against people of different races or ethnic groups.

Authenticity, then, offers no assurance of humaneness. And insincerity and hypocrisy needn't keep people from being kind, moral, or responsible. Some of the greatest political achievements, scientific breakthroughs, religious movements, and artistic creations have been initiated by people, who were mainly interested in promoting themselves, and who sometimes misrepresented their intentions or personal lives.

What the usual distinctions between authentic and inauthentic behavior also neglect to take into account is that the very process of socialization encourages the formation of public and private selves, as well as the development of certain social roles that rely on a degree of guile. If all people acted according to the dictates of their feelings, social intercourse would become chaotic and organized society couldn't exist. To live peacefully among others, people have to postpone instinctual gratifications and modify them for the public good. People who always shoot from the hip, take firm stands, speak their mind, and act according to their convictions may be admirable, but that usually only holds when we agree with them and they don't pose a threat to us.

And of course, just because people appear authentic doesn't mean they really are. People in certain professions actually may cultivate the appearance of sincerity because that is highly advantageous to them. Whenever people are trying to get other people to do something they may not be inclined to do, like buy certain products, vote in certain ways, or compromise their positions, a certain amount of manipulativeness and duplicity is often involved. As admirable a trait as authenticity may be, not too many businesspeople, salesmen, advertisers, diplomats, or politicians, with the rare exception of someone like Harry S. Truman, could thrive professionally if they were always true to their convictions and if they always said what they felt.

The notion of authenticity raises other problems, too. When authenticity can mean either being selfless or selfish, or becoming the person we can be versus simply being who we are, or even more common, a contradictory mixture of these, we encounter a confusing situation in which the hedonist who devotes his life to carnal pleasures can be just as authentic as the mystic who denies his flesh to gain transcendence.

In a sense, authenticity is very much a nineteenth- and early-twentieth-century notion, reflecting a certain view of human nature. It is a quaint but simplistic notion, which doesn't adequately explain the existence of mixed motivations, the unconscious determinants of behavior, and the rationalizations people use to justify what they do. Historically, it overlooks how rapid technological advances, information overload, mass communication media, and social complexity can affect the basic moral structure of people and how they view themselves. With all these changing social demands, which prompt the emergence of what Robert Lifton calls a "protean self," people may find it hard to retain a fixed identity along with a consistent set of values.[4]

Aside from these limitations, there is a more fundamental problem with the notion of authenticity: up until recent times, it has been mostly a "masculine" concept. The notion derives from Victorian times, when a man was taken at his word and business was transacted with a handshake. Being authentic was equivalent to being trustworthy and principled. It was the highest compliment you could pay another man. Authenticity was reserved mostly for men in privileged economic or social positions, who either followed a gentlemanly code of conduct or tried to live their lives according to the Good Book.

The fact that authenticity was seldom applied to women before the modern emphasis on "personal validation" as a way for women to affirm themselves, shows how biased this notion can be. In the past, women could be charming, graceful, talented, and even intelligent, but rarely authentic. You never concluded a deal with a woman on a handshake. The only way to assure a woman's trust was not through her morality but through her heart. As descendants of Eve, the temptress, women were assumed to be innately fickle and deceitful. But even if they weren't, another complication existed. Since women were the chattels of men or functioned in subsidiary roles, their word meant very little since they seldom had the final say. What good was it for them to be authentic when they commanded little social power and whatever they decided could be rescinded by their husbands, fathers, or guardians? When people are in a disadvantaged position and have little control over their own lives, they're more likely to resort to guile and cunning to achieve their goals than be perfectly frank with their oppressors about their intentions of manipulating them. Authenticity, then, can be a luxury, which the impoverished and oppressed can't afford. It also is a quality often reserved for heroes, who in the past mostly were men.

"Harry Truman was not a perfect man," David McCullough informed me. "He had very decided flaws, as we all do, and he made mistakes. But then that draws me to him, too. I'm not in the business of creating icons or heroic statues. I'm trying to tell the story of a life. . . . Form is everything. The form in this case is a straight-forward narrative. It begins at the beginning and it ends at the end, and it moves straight-forwardly

because he was a straight-forward sort of fellow. He was also, funda-
mentally, a nineteenth-century man. So the form is essentially like that
of a nineteenth-century life, like *David Copperfield*. And his question is,
as in *David Copperfield*, is he is going to turn out to be the hero of his
own story.

"And he does. It's a great American life. It's a great American story,
and I was drawn to Truman exactly because he is a great story. It's alle-
gorical, we see. He's Harry True Man. From a place called Independence,
the heart of America. And he goes off like Christian, in Bunyon's *Pil-
grim's Progress*, or any of the other great allegories, and he has his tests, his
adventures, one after another. There's an old adage about writing fiction
and drama, which is, 'Keep your hero in trouble.' Well, he's in trouble all
the time, and the question hangs, how's he going to get out of the hole?"
And it was a remarkable allegory, I think, how a man could have been
involved with the Pendergast political machine and still have retained his
personal integrity."

I expressed my skepticism to McCullough.

"I think he paid a price, and I think it shows in his headaches. He
had to check into the military hospital several times," he answered. "He
was under a great deal of stress because of the ethical strain on him. A lot
of this is revealed in his private journal entries. . . . There he tells us
candidly what's really been going on, and asks 'Did I do right?' That's
where he shows himself clearly in anguish.

"I'm often asked, 'How can Harry Truman, the man who desegre-
gated the armed services and sent the first civil rights message ever to
Congress, use words like "nigger" and "chink" and "kike?"' This reveals
him to be a fraud. In my view, historically, you should turn the question
around. The question is, how can a man, who grew up in an atmosphere
where words like 'nigger' and the rest were commonplace, turn out to be
the one who sends the first civil rights message to Congress and desegre-
gates the armed services? By the same token, I feel this kind of questioning applies to Truman's part in the Pendergast machine. Not so much
how can a fellow who seems to have such integrity have been involved
with an operation like that, but the reverse: How can someone who
came from that kind of a background have such integrity? That's what's

so astonishing. He survives that. He comes out of the swamp, and he comes out an exceptional politician. And I think you always have to use the word 'politician' because that was his career."

THE ILLUSION OF SELF-INVENTION

How do we reconcile the notion of authenticity with the modern emphasis on self-invention? Authenticity, by some accounts, means being who we are—expressing our innate dispositions and basic values—while self-invention means breaking free from the forces acting on us and assuming authorship for our life. Implicit in this notion of self-invention is the idea of ourselves as both Pygmalion and Galatea. Only limited by our natural endowments and circumstances, we supposedly have the power to transform ourselves into the person we hope to be. Almost any change is possible if we want it and work at it enough.

"In your book on Churchill, you talk about his being frail and small as a child and that he made a deliberate effort to make himself more pugnacious and audacious and courageous," I commented to William Manchester.

"He decided that biology is not destiny," he replied.

"You say he was one of the most authentic people you knew, in the sense that he was who he was in private as well as in public. And yet he is going against his biology or his inclinations. How do you reconcile that?"

"I think that it probably would have been impossible today. But the Victorian—and he was supremely Victorian—had absolute confidence in the individual's power to change himself and to meet whatever crisis came."

"Do you think this was deliberate on his part or was his response kind of sensed?"

"I don't see how it could have been deliberate, because it began when he was age seven. Other boys bullied him, and he hid in the woods. He decided that he would be the master of his fate, the captain of his soul."

"Is Teddy Roosevelt, in contrast to Truman, someone who invented himself?" I asked David McCullough, intrigued by Roosevelt's metamorphosis from a sickly youth to someone in robust health as an adult.

"I think Roosevelt is 'compensating' more for his own fears and his own sickly past and his own privileged upbringing, to be the kind of somebody he wanted to be. He wants to be a hero. He wants desperately to be out front, and he needs the limelight much more than Truman does. He has to have the limelight. He'll die without it. . . . And he is exceptionally gifted. He can do so many things. He has talent. Truman has no particular talent, at least as the culture judges talent. Roosevelt is a good writer. He's a good scholar. He has a phenomenal memory. He can speed read. He can read a whole book or two in a night and quote from it five years later. That's an exceptional man.

"Is he hiding things from himself and others?"

"Sure. More than even the rest of us."

"So if you had the opportunity of interviewing him, what would you want to know?"

"I don't think I'd get a word in edgewise. There are so many things. I would be interested in his interests, but I doubt that he would ever let me inside his emotional, private world. Here is a man who was the emblem of ebullient optimism and vigorous American confidence and all the rest, endlessly talkative and full of grand plans, who in his private life liked to sit alone in a room with the doors closed, reading Edwin Arlington Robinson, a poet of grief and despair. The fact that Theodore Roosevelt never even mentioned his first wife in his autobiography is what led me to think about writing about him. There's so much he's not telling us. And he always had a sense that he was a figure in history, that he is the hero of the drama. He's always very self-conscious about who he is, and that all eyes are on him and that he can amount to a lot in good part because of who he is."

Nowadays, the idea of self-invention is more than putting on a facade or acting in ways contrary to our background. With self-invention, we needn't fear being a phoney since, with our new narrative freedom, the person we create supposedly becomes us.[5] As "self-made" people, we have the potential to develop winning personalities, increase our brain power, become more sexually attractive, or compose our own life stories. We even have the option of fabricating authentic selves.

"Joshua Stanton," a friend of mine, illustrates this well. Born on a small farm in Kansas, he worked his way through college. After graduating, he spent a year at Oxford as a Rhodes scholar. When he returned to the States, he not only was a confirmed Anglophile but had become a staunch admirer of Winston Churchill, reading as many of his speeches and writings as he could as well as accounts of the monarchy and the lives of other prime ministers. Gifted with an almost photographic memory, he could come up with apt, often humorous quotes and aphorisms from this material to suit almost all occasions, and do so with the trace of an English accent and certain mannerisms of his hero. In time, he began dressing in English tweed, smoking occasional cigars, harrumphing when annoyed, and often seeking confrontations with colleagues over "principles," which then let him display his marvelous oratorical skills. Priding himself on his word, he developed a reputation for utter probity and for giving sage advice. Yet he had almost become a caricature of his idol, more Churchillian than Churchill himself, and as with Churchill, who also happened to invent himself, hardly ever deviated from his role, either in public or in private encounters. He was anything but genuine, yet in certain ways seemed more "authentic" than almost anyone I knew.

"Did Churchill see himself as hypocritical because of the demands of his public life?" I asked William Manchester.

"Churchill . . . needed a supporting cast to carry on what he was doing in his life," he responded. "Whether by luck or design, the woman he chose as his wife devoted her life to him, to the detriment of their children. . . . [He] also had certain advantages. He was a member of the British upper class. He never dressed himself. On one occasion he showed up at a villa on the Riviera, and when he arrived, he said to Maxine Elliot, 'I have traveled all the way from London without a valet.' And she murmured, 'Winston, how brave of you!' He seldom drove, which is fortunate, because he was a terrible driver. If he was in a traffic jam, he simply drove on the sidewalk. I think men who are going to achieve remarkable things have to perform in a way which is not really very admirable to the rest of the population."

"What distinguishes him from some of the other great people that we have known?"

"The fact that there was no difference whatever in Churchill delivering a major address and in Churchill in conversation."

What does all this tell us? It tells us that all the distinctions between "true" and "false" selves, or "authentic" and "inauthentic" selves, or "fulfilled" and "unfulfilled" selves make little sense, and have no basis in reality. All of these distinctions are based on the dubious assumption that there should be a congruence between our inner experiences and outer expressions, and that a harmonious relationship should exist among all components of the self, as supposedly happens in true, authentic, or fulfilled selves. But who decreed that this assumption be so? There is no reason why a Winston Churchill or a Teddy Roosevelt or a Katherine Mansfield or even my friend Josh should not be as authentic as a Harry Truman, if indeed, Truman was as genuine as he seemed. They simply are who they are, part revealed and part unrevealed, as Truman is, too. They may be more calculating or less straightforward, but their self-systems are just as real, and if we know enough about what went on in their minds and all the influences impinging upon them, their behavior would be as congruent with their motives, too.

The point is that everyone assumes certain roles and enters certain stories, but some of these roles and stories suit some people better than others. Being authentic is just as much a defined social role and part and parcel of certain kinds of life stories as being inauthentic. Certain expectations for behavior were inculcated in Truman by his parents, and the community in which he was raised happened to suit him well. Because of this fit, he didn't have to hide behind a public facade or invent himself anew as others with more conflicted and less stable self-systems had to do. But he may have had to if events had forced him to become a different version of himself.

Viewed in this light, the notions of self-invention and authenticity aren't incompatible. What we usually mean by an authentic self may simply be one that we happen to feel comfortable with, giving us little cause to seek another, and a reinvented self may simply express our desire to find another version of ourselves that suits us better. Because it derives from us, an invented self is just as genuine as any of our other creations. Even in multiple personality, the most dramatic instance of self-creation, we have no logical reason to assume that the alter personalities are any less genuine than the original one. But being genuine doesn't keep them from sometimes being unoriginal, shallow, or uninspired.

Do we, then, have the power to reinvent ourselves, to become, so to speak, plastic surgeons of our minds? Did Winston Churchill, for example, deliberately make up his mind at an early age to become more pugnacious and courageous, or did unseen forces induce him to choose this path? Did Rebecca, our imaginary heroine, really make an informed choice when she chose her mate, with the lifestyle that entailed, or did all her formative influences make her act as she did? Or in our case, when we adopt certain roles or assume a certain persona, do we do so intentionally, or is our choice shaped by drives we have little knowledge of?

How we answer these questions depends on whether we believe in free will. As potential masters of our fates, we have the capacity for self-invention; as fatalists, we don't. But the notion of self-invention poses special conceptual difficulties since we have a seemingly preposterous situation in which an insubstantial, hypothetical self undertakes the task of creating itself. Reminiscent of Escher's illusion of the creating hands, which seem to be operating independently of the original artist, the belief in self-invention requires that we remain ignorant of the forces that let us feel we have the power to create ourselves anew. To sustain an illusion of this sort, we must rely on complex mental maneuvers. Being aware of natural forces, we have to accept that whatever freedom we exert must be rooted in necessity, and being aware of our conscious thoughts and decisions, we have to experience the sense of free will in our very drivenness. This puts us in what appears to be an impossible predicament. But then, as we shall see, it reflects how our mind works.

ELEVEN

BIOGRAPHICAL
FREEDOM

THE FUNDAMENTAL QUESTION IS: How much control do you have over your life? Can you shape who you are or are you the inevitable product of multiple forces that shape you? Do you possess the narrative freedom to write your own life story or are you obliged to live out stories already written for you? Simply put, do you have freedom of choice or do you act out of necessity?

If you put aside the unlikely possibility that your mind can operate on some ethereal plane independent of your brain activity, then you're left to conclude that your mind and your brain must operate in concert and that mental events and neural events, though represented differently, are one and the same. All evidence supports this unitary position. For instance, electrical stimulation of different brain areas evokes different experiences. And different kinds of mental activity cause changes in cerebral blood flow and electrocortical activity. Now here is where the conceptual difficulties begin. The case for free will or determinism depends on which events initiate what. If neural events initiate thoughts and experiences, then your mental life must be based on strict physical causality, whether these neural events happen randomly or not. When physical causes are responsible for your mental activity, then you can't bear personal responsibility for your actions any more than a guided missile can bear responsibility for its. You act as you must. In contrast, if your thoughts can initiate neural activity, then you presumably can exert free will and assume responsibility for your actions as long as you identify your sense of "I" as the originator of these thoughts.

However, as we have seen before, whenever you invoke a phantom entity to explain the origination of a train of mental or neural events, you not only have to explain how this "prime mover" knows which of the billions of neurons to keep stimulating but also what factors are controlling it.[1] Quantum theory offers no solution to this problem. Regarding the brain as a probabilistic generator of thoughts still requires that you explain how certain of the random thoughts are selected. If you say that the control comes from within your mind, then you again need to conjure up the existence of an incorporeal mental guardian that decides which of these random thoughts to select. If you say that the control comes from outside you, then you create a Skinnerian scenario in which environmental factors mindlessly reinforce certain of your trial-and-error thought processes that are likely to lead to the most adaptive response.

Because the debate over free will and necessity remains unresolved, most explanatory systems of human behavior incorporate an immiscible mixture of both views. For example, while psychoanalytic theory holds that all mental experiences have antecedent causes, awareness of these causes supposedly frees up the person to exert control over them. Within many religious systems, believers are free to choose to follow the dictates of a Supreme Being who is the prime cause of all things. The teachings of Alcoholics Anonymous declare that alcoholics have no control over their drinking but can free themselves from their addiction by willingly conceding their helplessness and turning to a Higher Power for strength. Within the legal system, debate rages over the extent to which people are responsible for their crimes. The more accused people can blame their victims, society, inner passions, early abuses, or simply the absence of intention for their acts, the less likely they are to be held accountable for them. More and more, with this self-serving notion of causality, you can credit your free will with any decisions you make that suit you and blame any of your failings on the biological, psychological, or social forces operating on you.

What you find, then, is the tendency for people to rely on an oil-and-water concoction of free will and necessity to explain much of their personal and social behavior. But the reason for that, in my opinion, isn't because there are aspects of human behavior that can't be explained on the basis of either alone, but because of our deficient notions of psychological causality. The Newtonian notion of linear causality, whereby causes precede effects and actions lead to reactions, and the Pavlovian notion of classical conditioning, whereby specific stimuli elicit specific responses, and even quantum theory are inappropriate causal models for what transpires within the human mind.

To escape from the existing conceptual trap, you need to conceive of a causal system that doesn't require the presence of an originator—a homunculus—yet allows for flexible adjustments and choices to be made. A self-correcting, homeostatic self-system, which we discussed previously, represents such a model. Reminiscent of Gottfried Wilhelm von Leibniz's monads, which were centers of force or energy in which each state was a causal consequence of its preceding state, the self-system likewise seems to possess a "preestablished harmony" that is a guiding force for all change. But unlike Leibniz, the great seventeenth-century philosopher, you needn't invoke the existence of a divine originator to account for the genetic blueprints that guide your growth and development from the moment of your conception or for the cultural and environmental influences that modify their implementation. Whether a God or Nature is the architect behind these blueprints is irrelevant to the operation of this self-system. What is relevant is that these blueprints exist. The function of the self-system is to bring about compliance with these modifiable blueprints, while maintaining its own stability in the presence of constant flux and change. Within this unfolding causal system, every effect is implicit in every cause and every cause is implicit in every effect. Therefore, whatever freedom exists must be rooted in necessity, and whatever necessity exists must allow for the experience of personal choice.

I asked David McCullough how he made sense out of the person Teddy Roosevelt had become as an adult from the person he was as a child.

"What interested me was the metamorphosis, the transformation of the caterpillar to the butterfly, and what made that happen," he said. "How was it that this peculiar, frightened, sick, little boy with asthma turns into the emblem of American vitality and masculinity at the turn of the century? I was also experimenting with a form (in that book) that I hoped would be interesting, both from what it would reveal about the protagonist, and how it would turn out as a literary work. . . . In most biography, the main character is seen to grow and evolve into something else, the finished man or woman. That's the journey. His growth, his changing and developing, is the narrative, the story. And that is seen against . . . a cast of characters, who are nearly always given as fixed entities. They don't change. One of the reasons you see the main character change is because these other people are presented almost as stereotypes.

"But that isn't the way life is. It's important to understand everybody is changing, not just the main character, and particularly those people close to the main character who are having the greatest effect on his growth, his emotional and mental response to life.

"So in the case of Theodore Roosevelt, it isn't that you just have a certain kind of mother and a certain kind of father and a certain kind of sister and brother and so forth. How they are changing is affecting the main character. Sometimes they may even be changing much more dramatically than he. In the Theodore Roosevelt biography, I'm really writing biographies of five or six main characters, who in Roosevelt fashion, create a kind of swarm. They go everywhere together, they do everything together, and when Theodore really becomes himself, he breaks out of that. The close family world gives him both enormous confidence and saves his life when he's a sickly little fellow. But it's only when he breaks out of it—by getting into politics—that he emerges as his own man."

THE TERRITORY OF FREEDOM

There can be no sense of personal freedom that doesn't derive from your sense of "I." Your sense of "I" is predicated on awareness of your thoughts, experiences, and actions. Consciousness and the sense of freedom are intertwined. Yet probably more than 99.9 percent of your conscious activities require little effort of will. You do them out of habit, much as you drive a car over a long, straight stretch of road. You need no sense of "I" to make minor adjustments in your life that keep you on course and are consistent with your implicit plans and intentions. The self-system is most stable when all elements operate synchronously. When no glitches exist, nothing requires resolution, and when nothing needs resolution, you needn't exercise personal freedom. Your sense of "I" becomes most acute when adjustments within your self-system aren't automatic, such as when incompatibilities, problems, dilemmas, or ambiguities exist, and when you need to choose what strategies to adopt or which course to take.

As you shift from being less aware to being more aware of your thought processes, you simultaneously shift from a strictly deterministic mode of functioning, in which unconscious forces or conditioned responses govern your experiences, to a seemingly more volitional one, in which you initiate your own thoughts. What needs emphasis, though, is that the growing awareness of your thought processes doesn't change the actual nature of their causes, but only the way you interpret what is causing them and how responsible you feel for them. Just as the Schrödinger equation mathematically proved that the seemingly contradictory properties of light particles and waves were different manifestations of the same phenomenon, personal awareness of your mental processes serves as the equation that makes the seemingly contradictory properties of free will and necessity equivalent. When you aren't aware of the operation of your thought processes, you exist as an instinctive creature who responds as all brute animals do. Awareness lets you attribute personal volition to your thought processes and choices, although you remain ignorant of the multiple factors causing them.

The notion that awareness of certain events can make them seem different derives from Heisenberg's indeterminacy principle, which documents the influence of the observer on the observed event. Awareness of your thought processes transforms them from unaware-thought-processes to aware-thought-processes, which are the same yet not the same. Though the content of the unaware-thought-processes and aware-thought-processes may be identical, you experience the former as due to causal factors operating outside your control and the latter as being initiated by you. Because of constant shifts in your level of awareness, you shift from seeming to function as a machine to seeming to be in personal control.

Metaphorically, your self-system functions much like a symphony orchestra, with your sense of "I" serving as the conductor and the functions associated with the "me" as the instrumental sections. When the instrumental sections play harmoniously, the conductor loses himself in the melody, but when discordances, imprecisions, or missed notes arise, he suddenly becomes alert and acts to restore consonance. Whether the conductor's actions are deliberate or not has little to do with the entire orchestra's function, which is to play the assigned symphony as best it can. This is most likely to happen when all the musicians are receptive to the guidance of the conductor and when the conductor remains responsive to any deviations from the tune.

Free will and necessity, then, can be two sides of the same coin. You potentially become most free when you are aware of the discordances coming from the various instrumental sections within your mind and consciously can make adjustments that conform to the demands of your inner score, and you're least free when you get swept away by your performance or your thought processes remain unresponsive to the corrective actions of the "I." Stated differently, you have the psychological freedom to carry out the unfolding of your personal developmental blueprint, as constantly modified by the various influences impinging on you, and where inconsistencies or ambiguities exist, make adjustments that let you conform better to its essential motifs and leitmotifs or realize its full expression.

Where, then, is the territory of your freedom? The answer is simply that you're free whenever you are aware and not free whenever you are unaware of making a conscious decision. Your sense of efficacy grants you freedom, not what you actually do or think. Using chess as a metaphor, you can exercise free choice against an invincible opponent as long as you believe your decisions can alter the outcome of the game. Once you recognize that you have been forced into your moves, you no longer have a sense of personal freedom. You encounter a similar situation in real life. Ordinarily, you go about your daily activities without paying attention to the reasons for your ongoing thoughts and actions. When you encounter minor conflicts and incompatibilities, homeostatic mental mechanisms induce you to make corrective adjustments that will lead to a greater stability within your self-system. Most often, these automatic adjustments work. When they don't, you become aware that something is amiss. Unless you purposefully invoke it for self-reflection or problem-solving, awareness of your own mental processes usually represents a failure in the normal, homeostatic "housekeeping" activities of your self-system. It arises only when your typical repertoire of responses is insufficient to restore equilibrium within your self-system. It permits you to examine your situation and expand your range of options. Your deliberate selection of a particular response or your justification of it is what gives you your sense of personal freedom.

This brings up another matter. It isn't precise to say that you experience personal freedom when you become aware of choice. The qualifying point is that you also must feel that you have the power to implement that choice and move closer to realizing your goal. A self-correcting self-system only can gain equilibrium when a negative feedback loop exists. With this type of feedback loop, corrective adjustments are made to remedy deviations from the stable state.

Responses that are too great become dampened, and responses that are too muted become amplified. But as we've seen with many mental aberrations, positive feedback loops may take over when the self-correcting actions of the self-system break down. With this type of feedback loop, deviations from the stable state become perpetuated or worsened because responses that are too great become more amplified and responses that are muted become more dampened. Under these conditions, awareness of these breakaway mental processes only leads to a greater sense of helplessness and being out of control, and striving for inner harmony only leads to greater strife. To experience a sense of personal freedom, you have to take credit for any self-correcting adjustments within by your self-system that are designed to promote homeostasis as your personal life plan unfolds.

While your biological master plan is to pass through infancy, childhood, and adulthood on your way toward old age and death, your culture offers you a variety of modifiable myths and life stories to aid your transition through these obligatory phases. These myths and personal life stories establish the framework within which you can express what your genes and the modifying influences of your environment induce you to do. In most instances, continuous adjustments are necessary to allow a better fit between the personal life story you select or that is selected for you and your basic temperament and disposition. Within your unfolding, self-correcting self-system, which is geared toward optimal functioning and stability, you can attribute free will to any conscious efforts you make to bring your life in greater alignment with your life story or your personal life story in greater alignment with your natural inclinations.

As it happens, the narrator function of the "I" enhances your sense of free will. The very process of stringing together discrepant experiences in conformance to your implicit life story or aligning them with your underlying plans, myths, and inner schema, or engaging in the process of problem-solving, shifts the narrator function from a passive, subvocal observer to a more active commentator. As long as the story flow can continue unimpeded, you're not as likely to be aware of exerting choice. Your adjustments are spontaneous and fluid and don't require awareness. However, when you encounter obstacles, conflicts, or discrepancies, that's when you're apt to become most aware of the need for decisions and choices. The narrator function within your self-system swings into operation whenever your experiences get in the way of your doing what you're inclined to do. Because of homeostatic forces, the narrator function automatically works to resist any significant improvisations, digressions, and revisions of your implicit personal plot. It is this conscious experience of pursuing one course rather than another or solving certain problems or weighing options, all of which are designed to reestablish stability of your self-system, that enhances your sense of free will. Once your self-system is reequilibrated, you no longer have any need to be commenting inwardly on your experiences.

Some may object that it makes little sense to confine the sense of free will to acts designed to bring about optimal functioning of the self-system or a greater alignment of personal experiences with an implicit life story. If awareness of an experience is key to the sense of personal freedom, then this should hold for actions that are destabilizing to the self-system as well. This objection, however, contradicts what we already know about the operations of the mind. You're most likely to feel out of control or lacking in personal freedom when you can't shake off a depression or overcome an addiction or keep from overeating or rid yourself of obsessional thoughts. You don't deliberately try to make yourself miserable unless you want to expiate guilt, have masochistic inclinations, or are responding to obscure motives. This means that you essentially perceive all experiences or acts that lead to instability or suboptimal functioning of your self-system as due to destructive forces and not as exemplary of free will. You aren't apt to assume responsibility for any actions on your part that go contrary to your basic nature or substantially conflict with your life story. As certain psychological studies show, you're much more likely to take credit for positive outcomes than negative ones.[2] Unless seriously mentally disturbed or physically *in extremis*, you don't voluntarily choose to self destruct. The thoughts and actions you're most likely to take credit for are those that increase your sense of harmony, resonate with inner patterns, offer solutions to problems, or increase your feelings of personal agency. Just as metal filings arrange themselves within a magnetic field, you're most apt to experience personal freedom when you make conscious choices that reduce dissonance within yourself and that conform to the genetic, psychological, and cultural force fields in which you exist.

With this the case, you find that there is substantial slack within an unfolding causal system to let you operate with a sense of freedom. You can adopt strategies consistent with your unfolding genetic blueprint and personal life story that remove obstacles for personal growth, reduce distress, resolve conflicts, solve problems, enhance pleasure, and preserve health. You also can enjoy a degree of narrative freedom to reframe your life story when the plans and subplans that it must accommodate are inchoate, conflicting, or incomplete.

FREEDOM ROOTED IN NECESSITY

What I have been describing so far is a different notion of personal freedom, which is not only rooted in necessity but designed to facilitate it. It's an act of utter futility to rail against your fate, deny your biological inclinations, or disclaim your cultural heritage. You give up whatever freedom you possess by ignoring the reality of necessity. Swept along by a powerful current, you're least free to maneuver about in life when you futilely try to head upstream, and most free when your plans and actions are consistent with the flow of necessity.

The difficult dilemma you face, then, is how to maintain your sense of personal freedom while realizing that a myriad of unknown forces are controlling you. If you embrace the myth of free will, believing that you can be whatever you choose to be, you live your life oblivious to the many influences shaping your decisions. If you see yourself as the inevitable product of biological, psychological and cultural forces, completely lacking in choice, you deny your personal experience. Neither free will nor necessity fully captures the sense of who you are. Fortunately, there is a perspective that allows you considerable narrative freedom to construe your life as you see fit while acknowledging the inexorable forces impinging on you. Though subject to distortions, inaccuracies, and biases, a biographical perspective seems best suited among all the genres of composition for capturing your sense of self.

THE NATURE OF THE GENRE

What a biographical perspective tells you is that there are many ways to interpret your life, but that unlike fiction, you can't fabricate it out of whole cloth. The rules of the genre impose important constraints on you, the most important of which is verisimilitude. Far more limited than fiction writers, who can invent qualities or events to fit their preconceived image of a character, biographers work to bring about a fit between existing persons and all the existing information about them. Though this fit at times may seem as fanciful as a paleontolo-

gist's reconstruction of early humans and inferences about them from a few fragments of bone, the biographer, like the paleontologist, is obliged to take into
account the discovery of new artifacts and contrary evidence in the interpretation
of his or her subject.

"How do you really know someone?" I asked Victor Bockris. "How does
someone know you? If someone were to do a biography of you, would
they be likely to capture you? Would there be parts of you that would be
hidden?"

"It depends on what sort of access they have. If someone wrote
a biography of me and I agreed that person could talk to anyone I had
ever met and gave them the phone numbers and addresses of my old
girlfriends and my relatives, I think they could get a very good portrait. . . . What I'm saying is the perfect biography is possible. I'm
thinking about writing a biography of myself. But I emphasize the word
biography, not autobiography."

How, then, can you exert your biographical freedom? What exists is an abun-
dance of information about you that needs explanation and form. You have
potentially knowable but adumbrated parts of yourself that remain to be discovered and explored. By identifying the implicit plans and subplans that guide your
thoughts and govern your life, you gain the narrative freedom to move more
smoothly through your personal life story. When you realize better where you are
heading, you become more able to anticipate obstacles and weigh options for
adopting an alternative course.

Naturally, as an aspiring biographer of yourself, you must remain aware of
the limitations of your investigative tools. However impartial you try to be, your
observations always will be tainted by the nature of your perceptual apparatus,
the capacity of your brain, your biases, and your lack of access to crucial data
about yourself and the forces of Nature impinging on you. Because of this, you
may never have the foresight and capacity to fully compose the next chapter of
your life before you live it. But you still may know enough to be able to rough
out what it is likely to be if certain events happen and you respond to them in
certain ways.

ENTANGLED STORIES

As a social being, you can't function optimally without a basic understanding of the interpersonal system in which you exist. As much as you prefer to see yourself as autonomous and independent, others inhabit your life story and modify it in ways that may not be suitable to you. Even when you're alone, or dream, or fantasize, you carry important persons along in your head, some of whom—parents, teachers, supervisors, mentors, close friends, lovers—have a prominent place there. You constantly play to this unseen, mental audience, along with a faceless public, too, which sits in judgment of you.

Part of the limitations you face in fashioning a suitable narrative for yourself stems from your entanglement in other peoples' plots and the burden of having to play prescribed roles in their stories, which detract from what you otherwise prefer to do. These situations are familiar. An only daughter forgoes marriage and a career to devote much of her adult life to the care of her aging, hypochondriacal mother. Troubled parents argue constantly about how to handle their son, who is in constant trouble with the law, and use up most of their life savings in legal fees for his defense. A man grudgingly holds down two jobs in order to meet the mortgage payments for the expensive house his wife wants. Or a woman constantly puts aside her own wishes for a career to accommodate the expectations of her husband and children.

What this suggests is that whenever you're part of a unit of people, whether it be a couple, a family, a group, or a society, that unit exerts powerful influences on you, requiring you to incorporate it within your own life story and be responsive to its demands. This restricts your freedom to act within those areas of your life in which incompatibilities exist between others' expectations and yours. As a member of society, you never can escape these expectations entirely and are obliged to make certain accommodations to them. However, as in all personal actions, whether you regard your responses to the demands of others as voluntary depends on how aware of them you are. When you respond without conscious reflection or justification, you become an instinctive creature, obliged to act reflexively in certain ways to certain demands. When you remain aware of the mental processes associated with your responses, you are more apt to retain a feeling of personal choice. Even if your responses are obligatory or coerced, your telling yourself that you acted as you did because of expediency or realistic considerations increases your sense of autonomy by making you an active rather than passive participant in whatever happens to you. Whatever the reasons you give yourself for your actions, they imply that under different circumstances, you may have *chosen* to act otherwise.

> Harry Truman is exemplary of someone who could be independent yet also entangled in the lives of others.
>
> "He was a proud man . . . and proud of the fact that he had been a farmer," David McCullough said in response to my inquiry about how Truman might describe himself. "He was proud that he was a politician. He thought politics could be a noble profession. This is the old American idea, the farmer/politician, farmer/public servant, good citizen. He would probably call himself a 'citizen' in the old meaning of the word. He was a man of very strong affections. He truly adored his wife and his daughter. He adored his part of Missouri. He loved his country. I mean real love. I feel that his interest in the history of his country, for example, was an expression of his love. And he loved his mother, adored her. And he liked people. John Guenther once asked him, 'What are you really interested in?' And Truman said, 'People.' He thought that the most fascinating subject there is. Of course, he was right."

THE BIOGRAPHICAL SELF

You have no choice but to live your life within a biological format, proceeding inexorably from one life chapter to the next—from birth, to childhood, to adulthood, to death—but you needn't do so as a passive bystander in your unfolding, personal drama. A biographical perspective of yourself grants you the narrative freedom to shape the malleable aspects of your life. Most of your life story is implicit and ongoing, silently narrated or deftly perceived, but certain aspects await interpretation and definition. Your life, in a sense, represents a metaphor for its times, existing at a certain time and place in history, and exposed to the same infinitude of influences on others in a similar predicament. But as with any metaphor, it can be construed in many ways. While cultural myths and psychological needs shape your conception of yourself, you only gain the potential freedom to alter it when you can recognize the powerful forces that make you think as you do.

Although the biographical format obliges you to be rooted in reality (as you know it) and adopt a more objective perspective toward your self, it also gives you room to maneuver among the facts. Mostly, you live your life largely as you're disposed to and circumstances dictate, periodically constructing segues to help you get from where you are to where you want to be. You can't ignore important information about yourself, but as your own biographer, you can judge which material to select or ignore, what weight to place on it, whose opinions about you really matter, and what goals, themes, or plots run through your life. You also have the option to generate plausible explanations about yourself, the more imaginative the better. Although you never can be sure about the truth of your explanations, they remain plausible as long as they don't conflict with psychological, biological, and social reality. But the biographical genre also has its drawbacks. Since you never can have access to all the facts about you or understand the unfathomable aspects of your existence, any portrayal of you never can be complete. And since you also can't eliminate all autobiographical bias from your interpretation of the available information, other portrayals of you are possible, which may differ drastically from your own. Though you never can be sure that you are the entity you believe yourself to be, you nonetheless can take solace in one personal certainty. By adopting a biographical perspective of yourself, by definition, you become someone trying to make sense of who you are. It is during this very process of personal inquiry that you gain a heightened sense of your self-system, which represents your sense of "I" inextricably intertwined with your sense of "me." What Peer Gynt paradoxically never understood was that he was experiencing his self continuously all during his long and seemingly futile search. And that is as close as it's humanly possible to get to knowing who you truly are.

NOTES

PROLOGUE

I am indebted to all the biographers who generously agreed to be interviewed. Listed below are their names and the biographies they produced that have particular relevance to this project.

Christopher Benfey: *Emily Dickinson and the Problem of Others* (Amherst: University of Massachusetts Press, 1984); and *The Double Life of Stephen Crane* (New York: Alfred A. Knopf, 1992).

Victor Bockris: *Warhol* (London: Muller, 1989); *With William Burroughs: A Report from the Bunker* (New York: Seaver Books, 1981); *Lou Reed: The Biography* (London: Hutchinson, 1994); and *Keith Richards: The Biography* (New York: Poseidon Press, 1992).

Alan Bullock: *Hitler & Stalin: Parallel Lives* (New York: Alfred A. Knopf, 1992).

Humphrey Burton: *Leonard Bernstein* (New York: Doubleday, 1994).

James Collier: *Benny Goodman and the Swing Era* (New York: Oxford University Press, 1989); *Duke Ellington* (New York: Oxford University Press, 1987); and *Louis Armstrong: A Biography* (London: Michael Joseph, 1984).

Louise DeSalvo: *Virginia Woolf: The Impact of Childhood Sexual Abuse on Her Life and Work* (Boston: Beacon Press, 1989).

Scott Donaldson: *Archibald MacLeish: An American Life* (Boston: Houghton Mifflin, 1992); *Fool for Love: A Biography of F. Scott Fitzgerald* (New York: Delta, 1989); *By Force of Will: The Life and Art of Ernest Hemingway* (New York: The Viking Press, 1977); *John Cheever: A Biography* (New York: Random House, 1988); and *Poet in America: Winfield Townley Scott* (Austin: University of Texas Press, 1972).

Leon Edel: *Henry James: A Life* (New York: Harper and Row, 1985).

Charles Bracelen Flood: *Hitler: The Path to Power* (Boston: Houghton Mifflin, 1989); and *Lee: The Last Years* (Boston: Houghton Mifflin, 1981).

Peter Gay: *Freud: A Life for Our Time* (New York: Norton, 1988).

Brendan Gill: *Many Masks: A Life of Frank Lloyd Wright* (New York: G.P Putnam's Sons, 1987); *Lindbergh Alone* (New York: Harcourt, Brace, Jovanovich, 1977); and *Tallulah* (New York: Holt, Rinehart and Winston, 1972).

William Manchester: *The Last Lion: Winston Churchill, Vision of Glory, 1874–1932* (Boston: Little, Brown, 1983); *American Caesar: Douglas MacArthur, 1880–1964* (Boston: Little, Brown, 1978); and *H. L. Mencken: Disturber of the Peace* (New York: Collier, 1962).

David McCullough: *Truman* (New York: Simon and Schuster, 1992); and *Mornings on Horseback* (New York: Simon and Schuster, 1981).

Diane Middlebrook: *Anne Sexton: A Biography* (Boston: Houghton Mifflin, 1991).

Joan Peyser: *Bernstein: A Biography* (New York: William Morrow, 1987); and *The Memory of All That: The Life of George Gershwin* (New York: Simon and Schuster, 1993).

Arnold Rampersad: *The Art and Imagination of W. E. B. Du Bois* (Cambridge: Harvard University Press, 1976); *The Life of Langston Hughes: Volume I, 1902–1941: I, Too, Sing America* (New York: Oxford University Press, 1986); *The Life of Langston Hughes: Volume II, 1941–1967: I Dream a World* (New York: Oxford University Press, 1988); and *Days of Grace*, with Arthur Ashe, (New York: Knopf, 1993).

Roxana Robinson: *Georgia O'Keefe: A Life* (New York: Harper and Row, 1989).

Donald Spoto: *Marilyn Monroe: The Biography* (New York: HarperCollins, 1993); *The Dark Side of Genius: The Life of Alfred Hitchcock* (New York: Ballantine, 1983); *Laurence Olivier: A Biography* (New York: HarperCollins, 1992); *Blue Angel: The Life of Marlene Dietrich* (New York: Doubleday, 1992); and *The Kindness of Strangers: The Life of Tennessee Williams* (Boston: Little, Brown, 1985).

Wallace Stegner: *The Uneasy Chair: A Biography of Bernard DeVoto* (Garden City, NY: Doubleday, 1974).

Gloria Steinem: *Marilyn* (New York: Henry Holt, 1986).

Linda Wagner-Martin: *Sylvia Plath: A Biography* (New York: Simon and Schuster, 1987).

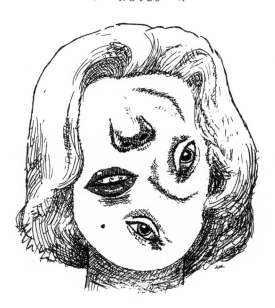

ONE: THE "REAL" MARILYN

1. For example, in a computerized literature search, I found only sixty-two biographies listed for John F. Kennedy and nineteen listed for Robert F. Kennedy.

2. The biographies I read are as follows: P. H. Brown and P. B. Barham, *Marilyn: The Last Take* (New York: Dutton, 1992); D. Conover, *Finding Marilyn: A Romance* (New York: Grosset and Dunlap, 1981); F. L. Guiles, *Legend: The Life and Death of Marilyn Monroe* (New York: Stern and Day, 1984); M. Haskell, *From Reverence to Rape: The Treatment of Women in the Movies* (New York: Holt, Rinehart and Winston, 1974); T. Jordan, *Norma Jean: My Secret Life with Marilyn Monroe* (New York: William Morrow, 1989); E. Hoyt, *Marilyn: The Tragic Venus* (Radnor, PA: Chilton Book Co., 1973); R. Kahn, *Joe & Marilyn: A Memory of Love* (New York: William Morrow, 1986); N. Mailer, *Of Women and Their Elegance* (New York: Simon and Schuster, 1980); N. Mailer, *Marilyn: A Biography* (New York: Grosset and Dunlap, 1973); G. McCann, *Marilyn Monroe* (New Brunswick, NJ: Rutgers University Press, 1988); J. Mellon, *Marilyn Monroe* (New York: Pyramid, 1973); A. Miller, *Timebends: A Life* (New York: Grove Press, 1987); J. Oppenheimer, *Marilyn Lives!* (New York: Delilah Books, 1981); R. Riese and N. Hitchens, *The Unabridged Marilyn: Her Life from A to Z* (New York: Congdon and Weed, 1987); D. Robinson and J. Kobal, *Marilyn Monroe: A Life on Film* (London: Hamlyn, 1974); C. E. Rollyson, Jr., *Marilyn Monroe: A Life of the Actress* (Ann Arbor: UMI Research Press, 1986); M. Rosen, *Popcorn Venus: Women, Movies and the American Dream* (New York: Coward, McCann and Geoghegan, 1973); N. Rosten, *Marilyn: An Untold Story* (New York: Signet, 1973); R. Slatzer, *The Life and Curious Death of Marilyn Monroe* (New York: Pinnacle, 1974); M. Speriglio, *The Marilyn Conspiracy* (New York:

Pocket Books, 1986); D. Spoto, *Marilyn Monroe: The Biography* (New York: HarperCollins, 1993); G. Steinem, *Marilyn* (New York: Henry Holt, 1986); S. Strasberg, *Marilyn and Me: Sisters, Rivals, Friends* (New York: Warner Books, 1992); A. Summers, *Goddess: The Secret Lives of Marilyn Monroe* (New York: Onyx Books, 1986); J. E. Wayne, *Marilyn's Men: The Private Life of Marilyn Monroe* (New York: St. Martin's Press, 1992); and M. Zolotow, *Marilyn Monroe* (New York: Harcourt, Brace, 1960).

3. Quoted in J. Mellon, *Marilyn Monroe*, 48.

4. Quoted in A. Miller, *Timebends*, 40–41.

5. See D. Spoto, *Marilyn Monroe: The Biography*.

6. Quoted in G. McCann, *Marilyn Monroe*, 31.

7. See my article, "Who Is Someone?" *American Journal of Psychotherapy*, 44 (1990): 516–24, for more details.

8. See H. Liebowitz, *Fabricating Lives: Explorations in American Autobiography* (New York: Alfred A. Knopf, 1989); P. J. Eakin, *Fictions in Autobiography: Studies in the Art of Self-Invention* (Princeton: Princeton University Press, 1985); D. C. Rubin, ed., *Autobiographical Memory* (London: Cambridge University Press, 1986); and S. Smith, "Constructing Truths in Lying Mouths: Truth-Telling in Women's Autobiography," *Studies in the Literary Imagination*, 23 (1990): 145–63, for in-depth discussions on the nature of autobiography.

9. M. Monroe, *Marilyn Monroe: My Story* (New York: Stein and Day, 1974).

10. M. Monroe, *Marilyn Monroe: My Story*, 194.

11. M. Monroe, *Marilyn Monroe: My Story*, 206.

12. N. Mailer, *Marilyn: A Biography*, 270.

13. D. Conover, *Finding Marilyn*, 151.

14. D. Robinson and J. Kobal, *Marilyn Monroe: A Life on Film*, 11.

15. W. Stegner, *Angle of Repose* (New York: Doubleday, 1971).

16. J. Givner, *Katherine Anne Porter: A Life* (New York: Simon and Schuster, 1982), 18.

17. E. S. Wolf, *Treating the Self: Elements of Clinical Self Psychology* (New York: Guilford Press, 1988).

18. D. Conover, *Finding Marilyn*, 186.

19. A. Miller, *Timebends*.

20. A. Summers, *Goddess: The Secret Lives of Marilyn Monroe*, 203.

21. Sharon O'Brien, "My Willa Cather: How Writing Her Story Shaped My Own," *New York Times Book Review*, February 20, 1994, 24.

22. *Diagnostic and Statistical Manual*, 4th ed., (Washington, D.C.: American Psychiatric Association, 1994).

23. A. Summers, *Goddess: The Secret Lives of Marilyn Monroe*, 307.

24. Marilyn Monroe has received many psychiatric diagnoses, ranging from depression to bipolar disorder and schizophrenia. In his book, *Goddess: The Secret Lives of Marilyn*

Monroe, Anthony Summers makes note that Dr. Valérie Shikverg, a consultant psychiatrist at several New York hospitals, believed that much of Monroe's behavior was consistent with borderline personality, and felt that this accounted for much of her behavior.

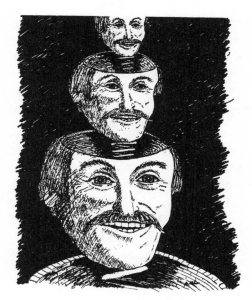

TWO: PEER GYNT'S ODYSSEY

1. See A.M. Ludwig, J. M. Brandsma, C. B. Wilbur, F. Bendfeldt, and D. H. Jameson, "The Objective Study of a Multiple Personality: Or, Are Four Heads Better Than One?" *Archives of General Psychiatry*, 26 (1972): 298–310.

2. See A.M. Ludwig, "Psychobiological Functions of Dissociation," *American Journal of Clinical Hypnosis*, 26 (1983): 93–99.

3. See K. J. Gergen, *The Saturated Self: Dilemmas of Identity and Contemporary Life* (New York: Basic Books, 1991).

4. H. Ibsen, *Peer Gynt*, J. W. McFarlane, ed., (London: Oxford University, 1970).

5. D. Middlebrook, *Anne Sexton: A Biography* (Boston: Houghton Mifflin, 1991), 62.

6. D. Middlebrook, *Anne Sexton: A Biography*, 349.

7. See R. B. Herberman, "Natural Killer Cells," *Hospital Practice*, April 1982: 93–103.

8. See D. C. Dennett, *Consciousness Explained* (Boston: Little, Brown, 1991), for an excellent discussion on the nature of our self boundaries and how they relate to bodily secretions and parts.

9. E. Hall, in *The Hidden Dimension* (Garden City, NY: Doubleday, 1969), describes a "critical distance" around each individual, a kind of psychological buffer zone, which

appears to have both biological and cultural roots. Individuals who violate the extended, personal body space of others usually elicit either fear or anger.

10. For discussions about how the architecture of the brain influences the sense of self, see R. W. Sperry, "Consciousness, Personal Identity, and the Divided Brain," in *The Dual Brain*, D. F. Benson and E. Zaidel, eds. (New York: Guilford, 1985); J. E. Bogen, "The Other Side of the Brain II: An Appositional Mind," *Bulletin of the Los Angeles Neurological Societies*, 34 (1969): 135–62; W. Penfield and T. Rasmussen, *The Cerebral Cortex of Man: A Clinical Study of Localization of Function* (New York: Hafner Publishing, 1968); W. Penfield and L. Roberts, *Speech and Brain-Mechanisms* (Princeton: Princeton University Press, 1959); K. R. Popper and J. C. Eccles, *The Self and Its Brain* (New York: Springer International, 1977); and L. W. Dewitt, "Consciousness, Mind, and Self: The Implications of the Split-Brain Studies," *British Journal for the Philosophy of Science*, 26 (1975): 41–60.

11. The following sources offer excellent overviews of different theories and issues about the nature of the self: R. F. Baumeister, *Meanings of Life* (New York: Guilford, 1991); R. F. Baumeister, *Identity: Cultural Change and the Struggle for Self.* (New York: Oxford University Press, 1986); K. J. Gergen, *The Concept of the Self* (New York: Holt, Rinehart and Winston, 1971); J. D. Levin, *Theories of the Self* (Washington: Hemisphere Publishing, 1992); B. R. Schlenker, ed., *The Self and Social Life* (New York: McGraw-Hill, 1985); and M. Rosenberg, *Conceiving the Self* (New York: Basic Books, 1979).

12. Abbé de Condillac, *Philosophical writings of Etienne Bonnot, Abbé de Condillac*, trans. F. Philip (Hillsdale, NJ: Lawrence Erlbaum Assoc. Publishers, 1982).

13. See J. D. Levin, *Theories of the Self*, for in-depth reviews of these theories.

14. See J. D. Levin, *Theories of the Self.*

15. See William James's brilliant discussion of the concept of self in his *Principles of Psychology* (New York: Henry Holt, 1950).

16. Julian Jaynes's *The Origin of Consciousness in the Breakdown of the Bicameral Mind* (Boston: Houghton Mifflin, 1976) offers an original but highly speculative account about the importance of recorded language and the narrative process for the development of the self.

17. J. F. Masterson (*The Search for the Real Self: Unmasking the Personality Disorders of Our Age* [New York: Free Press, 1988]), for example, claims that the false self is inhibited and conflictual and the true self is liberated of its inhibitions by psychotherapy. Also see J. T. Tedeschi, "Private and Public Experiences and the Self," in R. F. Baumeister, ed., *Public Self and Private Self* (New York: Springer-Verlag, 1986); R. D. Laing, *Self and Others* (New York: Penguin Books, 1969); R. D. Laing, *The Divided Self* (New York: Pantheon Books, 1960); B. R. Schlenker, "Self-Identification: Toward an Integration of the Private and Public Self," in. R. F. Baumeister, ed., *Public Self and Private Self*; L. Josephs, *Character and Structure and the Organization of the Self* (New York: Columbia

University Press, 1992); R. F. Baumeister and D. M. Tice, "Four Selves, Two Motives, and a Substitute Process Self-Regulation Model," in R. F. Baumeister, ed., *Public Self and Private Self*, and the important conceptual article by S. Epstein, "The Self-Concept Revisited: Or a Theory of a Theory," *American Psychologist*, May 1973: 404–16.

18. See R. Schaffer, *Retelling a Life: Narration and Dialogue in Psychoanalysis* (New York: Basic Books, 1992) and L. Rue, *By the Grace of Guile: The Role of Deception in Natural History and Human Affairs* (London: Oxford University Press, 1994) for an interesting analysis of self-deception. Rue argues against self-deception being paradoxical. He claims that if the role of the self is to devise strategies of behavior to eliminate or inhibit potentially conflicting instructions, some deception of others is advantageous from an evolutionary perspective. However, since it likewise is biologically advantageous for others to learn ways to perceive deception, the best solution is for a person to believe his own lies so that he doesn't give off telltale signs.

19. A. N. Whitehead, *Process and Reality* (New York: Macmillan, 1929) and *Adventures of Ideas* (New York: Free Press, 1933).

20. Also see M. Csikszentmihalyi, *The Evolving Self: A Psychology for the Third Millennium* (New York: HarperCollins, 1993); M. Lewis and J. Brooks-Gunn, *Social Cognition and the Acquisition of Self* (New York: Plenum Press, 1979); J. Kagan, *Unstable Ideas: Temperament, Cognition, and Self* (Cambridge: Harvard University Press, 1989); E. H. Erikson, *Childhood and Society* (New York: W. W. Norton, 1950); E. H. Erikson, *The Life Cycle Completed* (New York: W. W. Norton, 1982); and R. M. Galatzer-Levy and B. J. Cohler, *The Essential Other: A Developmental Psychology of the Self* (New York: Basic Books, 1993).

21. For a sampling of the ways different cultures view the self, see Alan Roland, *In Search of Self in India and Japan* (Princeton: Princeton University Press, 1988); Sudhir Kakar, "Western Science, Eastern Minds," *The Wilson Quarterly*, Winter, 1991: 109–16; M. R. Markus and S. Kitayama, "Culture and the Self: Implications for Cognition, Emotion and Motivation," *Psychological Review*, 98 (1991): 224–53; Michelle Z. Rosaldo, "Toward an Anthropology of Self and Feeling," in R. A. Shweder and R. A. Levine, eds., *Culture Theory* (Cambridge: Cambridge University Press, 1984); C. Geertz, "'From the native's point of view' on the Nature of Anthropological Understanding," in R. A. Shweder and R. A. LeVine, eds., *Culture Theory* (Cambridge: Cambridge University Press, 1984); and A. M. Ludwig, "Culture and Creativity," *American Journal of Psychotherapy*, 46 (1992): 454–69.

22. R. A. Shweder and E. J. Bourne, "Does the Concept of the Person Vary Cross-Culturally?" In R. A. Shweder and R. A. LeVine, eds., *Culture Theory*.

23. See C. F. Cooley, *Human Nature and the Social Order* (New York: Scribner, 1902), and G. H. Meade, *Mind, Self, and Society from the Standpoint of a Social Behavioralist* (Chicago: University of Chicago Press, 1934). Also see J. D. Levin, *Theories of the Self*

(Washington, D. C.: Hemisphere Publishing, 1992), for a discussion of this topic.

24. See E. Auerbach, *Mimesis* (Princeton: Princeton University Press, 1991); R. Whittemore, *Pure Lives: The Early Biographers* (Baltimore: The Johns Hopkins University Press, 1988); R. Whittemore, *Whole Lives: Shapers of Modern Biography* (Baltimore: The John Hopkins University Press, 1989); K. J. Weintraub, *The Value of the Individual: Self and Circumstance in Autobiography* (Chicago: University of Chicago Press, 1978); R. F. Baumeister, *Identity: Cultural Change and the Struggle for Self* (New York: Oxford University Press, 1986); and P. Cushman, *Constructing the Self, Constructing America: A Cultural History of Psychotherapy* (Reading, MA: Addison-Wesley Publishing, 1995), for excellent discussions of the changing notions of the self throughout history in fiction and biography.

25. V. Woolf, *Orlando: A Biography* (New York: Crosby Gaige, 1928).

26. N. Mailer, *Of Women and Their Elegance* (New York: Simon and Schuster, 1980), and N. Mailer, *Marilyn: A Biography* (New York: Grosset and Dunlap, 1973).

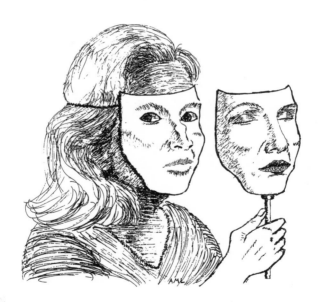

THREE: MASQUERADE

1. See L. Funderburg, *Black, White, Other: Biracial Americans Talk About Race and Identity* (New York: William Morrow, 1994), for how this dilemma especially affects biracial individuals.

2. R. Ellison, *Invisible Man* (New York: Vintage Books, 1989), 577.

3. K. Douglas, *The Ragman's Son* (New York: Simon and Schuster, 1988).

4. E. Goffman, in his pioneer work, *Stigma* (Englewood Cliffs, NJ: Prentice Hall,

1963), offers a penetrating analysis of the impact of all varieties of social stigmas on the behaviors and lives of those afflicted. Most of my observations on this topic have been anticipated by him.

5. There is an extensive literature on impression management and image manipulation. Again, Erving Goffman has written a classical work in this field, entitled, *The Presentation of Self in Everyday Life*, Monograph 2 (Edinburgh: University of Edinburgh, Social Science Research Centre, 1958). Also see E. Jones and T. S. Pittman's review chapter on this topic, "Toward a General Theory of Strategic Self-Presentation," in *Psychological Perspectives on the Self*, vol. 1, Jerry Suls, ed., (Hillsdale, NJ, Lawrence Erlbaum Associates, 1982).

6. R. E. Park, *On Social Control and Collective Behavior: Selected Papers* (Chicago: University of Chicago Press, 1967); R. E. Park, *Race and Culture* (Glencoe, IL: The Free Press, 1950).

7. S. de Beauvoir, *The Second Sex*, trans. H. M. Parshley (New York: Knopf, 1953).

8. A. Ashe and A. Rampersad, *Days of Grace* (New York: Knopf, 1993), 127.

9. A. Ashe and A. Rampersad, *Days of Grace*, 138.

10. E. Goffman, *Stigma*.

11. E. Goffman, *Stigma*.

12. See G. Clark, *Capote: A Biography* (New York: Simon and Schuster, 1988); C. House, *The Outrageous Life of Henry Faulkner* (Knoxville: The University of Tennessee Press, 1988); and R. Ellman, *Oscar Wilde* (New York: Alfred A. Knopf, 1988).

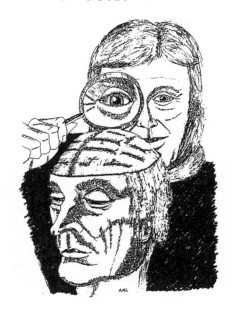

FOUR: EXISTING ON DIFFERENT PLANES

1. J. Cheever, *The Journals of John Cheever* (New York: Alfred A. Knopf, 1991), 232.

2. A. M. Ludwig, "Who is Someone?" *American Journal of Psychotherapy*, 44 (1990): 516–24.

3. See W. M. Runyan, *Psychology and Historical Interpretation* (New York: Oxford University Press, 1988), for discussion of the relationship of plausibility to biographical truth.

4. W. M. Runyan, *Psychology and Historical Interpretation* (New York: Oxford University Press, 1988).

5. L. G. Sexton, *Searching for Mercy Street: My Journey Back to My Mother, Anne Sexton* (Boston: Little, Brown, 1994).

6. R. Robinson, *Georgia O'Keefe: A Life* (New York: Harper and Row, 1989).

7. See R. F. Baumeister, *Identity: Cultural Change and the Struggle for the Self* (New York: Oxford University Press, 1986) and M. Rosenberg, *Conceiving the Self* (New York: Basic Books, 1979), for excellent discussions on the importance of labels for establishing personal identity.

8. A. G. Greenwald, "The Totalitarian Ego: Fabrication and Revision of Personal History," *American Journal of Psychology*, 35 (1980): 603–18.

9. R. F. Baumeister, *Identity: Cultural Change and the Struggle for the Self*.

10. J. B. Chassan, *Research Design in Clinical Psychology and Psychiatry* (New York: Appleton-Century-Crofts, 1967).

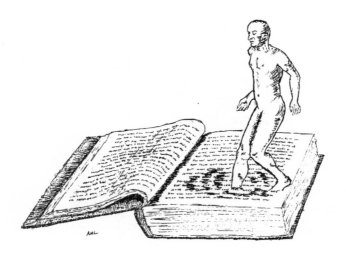

FIVE: LIVING BACKWARDS

1. C. Benfey, *The Double Life of Stephen Crane* (New York: Knopf, 1992).

2. J. Kagan, *Galen's Prophesy: Temperament in Human Nature* (New York: Basic Books, 1994). Also see W. Gallagher, "How We Become What We Are," *The Atlantic Monthly*, September 1994, 39–55; and C. R. Cloninger, D. M. Svrakic, and T. R. Przybeck, "A Psychological Model of Temperament and Character," *Archives of General Psychiatry*, 50 (1993): 975–90.

3. See M. Csikszentmihalyi and O. V. Beattie, "Life Themes: A Theoretical and Empirical Exploration of Their Origins and Effects," *Journal of Humanistic Psychology*, 19 (1979): 45–63, for how unresolved, early life conflicts have profound effects on the dominant themes governing individual's lives. Of course, this is likewise a basic assumption of psychoanalytic theory.

4. See J. Campbell, *The Power of Myth*, with B. Moyers (New York: Doubleday, 1988) and J. Campbell, *The Hero with a Thousand Faces* (Princeton: Princeton University Press, 1968). Also see S. Keen and A. Valley-Fox, *Your Mythic Journey: Finding Meaning in Your Life Through Writing and Storytelling* (Los Angeles: Jeremy P. Tarcher, 1989); L. Rue, *By the Grace of Guile: The Role of Deception in Natural History and Human Affairs* (London: Oxford University Press, 1994); and D. P. McAdams, *The Stories We Live By: Personal Myths and the Making of the Self* (New York: William Morrow, 1993) for discussions of the role of myths and stories in our lives.

5. Plots can be driven by talent or intellectual and motivational needs as well. By virtue of a superior facility, a person can be drawn to art, music, or chess as a major medium for personal expression and then, eventually, for personal fulfillment. Gerald Holton, in *Thematic Origins of Scientific Thought: Kepler to Einstein* (Cambridge: Harvard University Press, 1973), describes the importance of "themata," around which individuals organize

their lives and ideas. Also see E. E. Jones, "Interpreting Interpersonal Behavior: The Effects of Expectancies," *Science*, 234 (1986): 41–46 for an excellent account of the role of expectancies in human behavior. A. G. Greenwald, "The Totalitarian Ego: Fabrication and Revision of Personal History," *American Journal of Psychology* 35 (1980): 603–18, discusses the reasons for cognitive constancy.

6. There is vast literature on social role therapy. Talcott Parsons, of course, has written the pioneer work in this area. See *The Social System* (Glencoe, IL: Free Press, 1959). Also see D. P. McAdams, *The Stories We Live By: Personal Myths and the Making of the Self*, and R. F. Baumeister, *Identity: Cultural Change and the Struggle for the Self* (New York: Oxford University Press, 1986).

7. P. Evans, *Peter Sellers: The Mask Behind the Mask* (Englewood Cliffs, NJ: Prentice-Hall, 1968), 191.

8. D. Spoto, *Laurence Olivier: A Biography* (New York: HarperCollins, 1992), 290.

9. D. Spoto, *Laurence Olivier*, 377.

10. D. P. McAdams (*The Stories We Live By: Personal Myths and the Making of the Self*) discusses the importance of "imagoes" and role models in our lives.

11. Silvan S. Tomkins ("Script Theory," in *The Emergency of Personality*, J. Aronoff, A. I. Rabin, and Robert A. Zucker, eds., [New York: Springer Publishing, 1987]) also developed an important theory about human behavior based on "scripts." In his particular usage of the term, a script represents the basic unit of analysis for understanding persons. Some scripts are innate, but most are innate and learned. The learned scripts originate in innate scripts but usually radically transform them. These innate and learned scripts, in turn, affect most behavior patterns in adult life. Also see M. J. Horowitz, "Person Schemas," in *Person Schemas and Maladaptive Interpersonal Patterns*, M. J. Horowitz ed., (Chicago: University of Chicago Press, 1991); J. L. Singer and P. Salovey, "Organized Knowledge Structures and Personality: Person Schemas, Self Schemas, Prototypes, and Scripts," in *Person Schemas and Maladaptive Interpersonal Patterns*, M. J. Horowitz, ed.

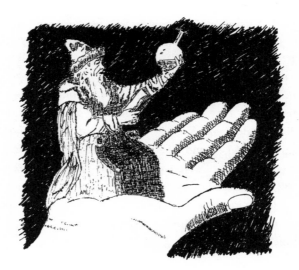

SIX: THE PHILOSOPHER'S STONE

1. Lexington *Herald-Leader*, September 17, 1992.

2. Lexington *Herald-Leader*, August 7, 1994.

3. *Newsweek*, Deecember 2, 1996.

4. R. Price, *A Whole New Life* (New York: Atheneum, 1994).

5. J. Weimer, *Back Talk: Teaching Lost Selves to Speak* (New York: Random House, 1994).

6. Lexington *Herald-Leader*, March 1, 1996.

7. See D. P. McAdams, *The Stories We Live By: Personal Myths and the Making of the Self* (New York: William Morrow, 1993) and J. Campbell, *The Power of Myth*, with Bill Moyers, (New York: Doubleday, 1988). Also see L. Rue, *By the Grace of Guile: The Role of Deception in Natural History and Human Affairs* (London: Oxford University Press, 1994).

8. Jules Masserman (*The Practice of Dynamic Psychiatry* [Philadelphia: W. B. Saunders, 1955]) describes three basic Ur-defenses of man that border on the delusional. The first Ur-defense is the delusion of invulnerability and immortality, the components of which include the belief in an absence of personal threat, the persistence of self, and the power to control the outside world. The second Ur-defense is the delusion of the omnipotent servant, whereby certain individuals become ordained with a divine-like power to heal others and to communicate with the gods. The third Ur-defense pertains to the belief in man's kindness to man, the notion that in time of need one can seek and actually obtain success from one's fellow man.

Shelley E. Taylor (*Positive Illusions: Creative Self-Deception and the Healthy Mind* [New York: Basic Books, 1989]) claims that a healthy mind is self-deceptive in that it creates beneficent interpretations of threatening events that raise self-esteem and promote motivation. The self revises and fabricates personal history through self-enhancement, exaggerated beliefs in personal control, and unrealistic optimism. Lauren B. Alloy reports that depressives are far more realistic about their ability to control uncontrollable but satisfying outcomes than people who are mentally healthy; in contrast, they are more apt to believe wrongly that others have the power to increase a good experimental outcome ("Depressive Realism: Sadder but Wiser?" *The Harvard Mental Health Letter*, April, 1995). F. Rothbaum, J. R. Weisz, and S.S. Snyder, "Changing the World and Changing the Self: A Two-Process Model of Perceived Control," *Journal of Personality and Social Psychology*, 42 (1982): 5–37, claim that people try to gain control not only by bringing the environment in line with their primary wishes but by bringing themselves in line with environmental forces. They do this by trying to gain interpretive control over otherwise uncontrollable events.

9. See S. E. Taylor, *Positive Illusions: Creative Self-Deception and the Healthy Mind* (New York: Basic Books, 1989) and M. White and D. Epston, *Narrative Means to Therapeutic Ends* (New York: W. W. Norton, 1990).

10. R. F. Baumeister (*Meanings of Life* [New York: Guilford, 1991]) has written one of the most thoughtful and impressive books on the importance of meaning in our lives. I'm indebted to him for his observations on this topic.

11. A. Wheelis, *Quest for Identity* (New York: W. W. Norton, 1966).

12. See C. R. Snyder and H. L. Fromkin, eds., *Uniqueness: The Human Pursuit of Difference* (New York: Plenum, 1980).

13. See R. F. Baumeister, *Meanings of Life*.

14. Quoted by V. Frankl, *Man's Search for Meaning: An Introduction to Logotherapy* (New York: Washington Square Press, 1963).

15. A. Wheelis (*Quest for Identity*) describes this basic existential dilemma well.

16. S. Beckett, *Waiting for Godot* (New York: Grove Press, 1954).

17. V. Frankl, *Man's Search for Meaning*.

18. See C. S. Carter, "Oxytocin and Sexual Behavior," *Neuroscience Biobehavioral Review*, 16 (1992): 131–34; T. R. Insel, "Oxytocin, A Neuropeptide for Affiliation: Evidence from Behavioral, Receptor Autoradiographic, and Comparative Studies," *Psychoendocrinology*, 17 (1992): 3–33; and T. R. Insel and T. J. Hulihan, "A Gender-Specific Mechanism for Pair Bonding: Oxytocin and Partner Preference Formation in Monogamous Voles," *Behavioral Neuroscience*, 109 (1995): 782–89.

19. See A. Mazur, "A Cross-Species Comparison of Status in Small Established Groups," *American Sociological Review*, 38 (1973): 513–30, for a description of deference behavior in higher primates. Also see M. R. A. Chance and C. J. Jolly, *Social Groups of Monkeys, Apes, and Men* (London: Jonathan Cape, 1970); R. I. M. Dunbar, *Primate Social Systems* (New York: Cornell University Press, 1988); D. Fossey, *Gorillas in the Mist* (Boston:

Houghton Mifflin, 1983); E. O. Wilson, *Sociobiology* (Cambridge: Harvard University Press, 1980); J. Goodall, *The Chimpanzees of Gombe: Patterns of Behavior* (Cambridge: Harvard University Press, 1986); R. A. Heifetz, *Leadership Without Easy Answers* (Cambridge: Harvard University Press, 1994); and F. de Waal, *Chimpanzee Politics: Power and Sex Among the Apes* (London: Jonathan Cape, 1982).

20. R. M. Sapolsky ("Hypocortisolism Among Socially Subordinate Wild Baboons, *Archives of General Psychiatry*, 46 [1989]: 1047–51) has documented biochemical changes in baboons induced by changes in their social status.

21. M. Wollstonecraft, *A Vindication of the Rights of Women* (New York: W. W. Norton, 1975), 34.

22. M. Wollstonecraft, *A Vindication of the Rights of Women*, 20.

23. J. V. Craig, *Domestic Animal Behavior: Causes and Implications for Animal Care and Management* (Englewood Cliffs, NJ: Prentice-Hall, 1981); I. L. Mason, ed., *Evolution of Domesticated Animals* (London: Longman, 1984); and S. Budzansky, *The Covenant of the Wild: Why Animals Chose Domestication* (New York: William Morrow, 1992).

24. See S. Budzansky, *The Covenant of the Wild*, for a fascinating account of neoteny and his theories about the nature of domestication.

25. S. J. Gould, "A Biological Homage to Mickey Mouse," in *The Panda's Thumb: More Reflections in Natural History* (New York: W. W. Norton, 1980), 95–107.

26. E. Becker, *Denial of Death* (New York: The Free Press, 1973). Also see E. Becker, *Escape From Evil* (New York: The Free Press, 1975).

27. A. M. Ludwig, "Altered States of Consciousness," *Archives of General Psychiatry*, 15 (1966): 562–68.

28. W. James, *Varieties of Religious Experience* (New York: Modern Library, 1929).

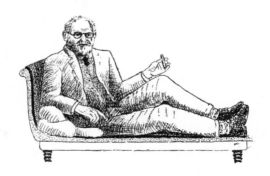

SEVEN: PSYCHOANALYZING FREUD

1. A. M. Ludwig, J. Levine, and L. H. Stark, *LSD and Alcoholism: A Study of Treatment Efficacy* (Springfield, IL: Charles C. Thomas, 1970).

2. S. Freud, "Analysis of a Phobia in a Five Year Old Boy," in *Sigmund Freud: Collected Papers*, vol. 3, trans. A. Strachey and J. Strachey (New York: Basic Books, 1959).

3. See J. Wolpe and S. Rachman ("Psychoanalytic 'Evidence': A Critique Based on Freud's Case of Little Hans," *Journal of Nervous and Mental Disease*, 131 [1960]: 135–48) for a comparison of psychoanalytic to a behavioral understanding of Little Hans's difficulties.

4. J. A. V. Galvin and A. M. Ludwig, "A Case of Witchcraft," *The Journal of Nervous and Mental Disease*, 133 (1961): 161–68.

5. What little prior research that has been done on the relative effectiveness of different theoretical persuasions suggests that they all display comparable efficacy in the hands of skilled practitioners. See J. Frank, *Persuasion and Healing* (Baltimore: Johns Hopkins Press, 1961); L. Luborsky, B. Singer, and L. Luborsky, "Comparative Studies of Psychotherapies: Is It True That Everyone Has Won and All Must Have Prizes?" *Archives of General Psychiatry*, 32 (1975): 995–1008; H. J. Eysenck, "The Effects of Psychotherapy: An Evaluation," *Journal of Consulting Psychology*, 16 (1952): 319–24, 1952; and D. H. Ford and H. B. Urban, *Systems of Psychotherapy: A Comparative Study* (New York: John Wiley and Sons,1965).

6. See P. Gay, *Freud: A Life for Our Time* (New York: W. W. Norton, 1988), and E. Jones, *The Life and Work of Sigmund Freud*, vols. 1–3, (New York: Basic Books, 1953).

7. See J. M. Masson, *The Assault on Truth: Freud's Suppression of the Seduction Theory* (New York: Farrar, Straus, and Giroux, 1984).

8. See A. Huxley, *The Devils of Loudun* (London: Chatto and Windus, 1952); M. Summers, *The History of Witchcraft and Demonology* (New York: University Books, 1956); and *Malleus Malleficarum*, trans. and intro. by M. Summers, (London: Pushkin Press, 1951).

9. P. Gay, *Freud: A Life for Our Time*.

10. D. P. Spence, *Narrative Truth and Historical Truth: Meaning and Interpretation in Psychoanalysis* (New York: Norton, 1982).

11. For further descriptions of the role of narrative in psychotherapy, see L. Sheingold, *Soul Murder* (New Haven, CT: Yale University Press, 1989); P. R. McHugh and P. R. Slavney, *The Perspectives of Psychiatry* (Baltimore: The Johns Hopkins University Press, 1983); M. White and D. Epston, *Narrative Means to Therapeutic Ends* (New York: W. W. Norton, 1990); G. S. Howard, "Culture Tales: A Narrative Approach to Thinking, Cross-Cultural Psychology, and Psychotherapy," *American Psychologist*, 46 (1991): 187–97; and R. Schaffer, *Retelling a Life: Narration and Dialogue in Psychoanalysis* (New York: Basic Books, 1992).

12. J. Cheever, The Journals of John Cheever (New York: Knopf, 1991), 156.

13. D. Middlebrook, *Anne Sexton: A Biography* (Boston: Houghton Mifflin, 1991).

14. D. Middlebrook, (1991). *Anne Sexton*, 56.

15. D. Middlebrook, (1991). *Anne Sexton*, 63.

16. D. Middlebrook, (1991). *Anne Sexton*, 62.

17. D. Middlebrook, (1991). *Anne Sexton*, 64.

18. A. M. Ludwig, "The Formal Characteristics of Therapeutic Insight," *American Journal of Psychotherapy*, 20 (1966): 305–18.

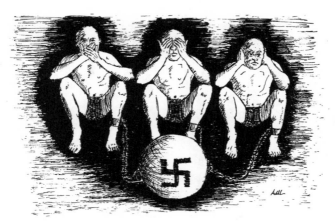

EIGHT: HOW DID HITLER LIVE WITH HIMSELF?

1. See A. Delbanco, *The Death of Satan* (New York: Farrar, Straus, and Giroux, 1995) for an excellent overview of the role of evil in Western civilization.

2. A. Bullock, *Hitler & Stalin: Parallel Lives* (New York: Alfred A. Knopf, 1992).

3. C. B. Flood, *Hitler: The Path to Power* (Boston: Houghton Mifflin, 1989).

4. Quoted in D. J. Hershman and J. Lieb, *A Brotherhood of Tyrants: Manic Depression and Absolute Power* (Amherst, NY: Prometheus Books, 1994), 152.

5. Quoted in D. J. Hershman and J. Lieb, *A Brotherhood of Tyrants*, 182.

6. M. Burleigh, *Death and Deliverance: 'Euthanasia' in Germany c. 1900–1945* (Cambridge: Cambridge University Press, 1994).

7. M. Burleigh, (1994). *Death and Deliverance*, 191.

8. M. Burleigh, (1994). *Death and Deliverance*, 274–75.

9. M. Burleigh, (1994). *Death and Deliverance*, 275.

10. R. J. Lifton, *The Nazi Doctors* (New York: Basic Books, 1982).

11. H. Arendt, *Eichmann in Jerusalem: A Report on the Banality of Evil* (New York: Viking Press, 1963).

12. See R. F. Baumeister, *Meanings of Life* (New York: Guilford, 1991).

13. S. Milgram, *Obedience to Authority* (New York: Harper and Row, 1974).

14. Lexington *Herald-Leader*, November 3, 1994.

15. R. J. Lifton, *The Nazi Doctors*, 501.

16. R. C. Tucker, "A Stalin Biographer's Memoir," in *Introspection in Biography: A*

Biographer's Quest for Self-Awareness, S. H. Baron and C. Pletsh, eds., (Hillside, NJ: Analytic Press, 1985), 266.

17. R. C. Tucker, "A Stalin Biographer's Memoir," 265.

18. R. C. Tucker, "A Stalin Biographer's Memoir," 270.

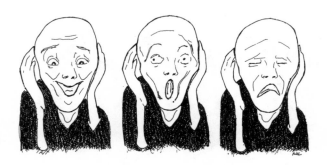

NINE: WHAT MADNESS REVEALS

1. See T. Leary, *Neuropolitics: The Sociobiology of Human Metamorphosis* (Los Angeles: A Starseed/Peace Press Publication, 1977).

2. R. D. Laing, *The Politics of Experience* (New York: Pantheon, 1967).

3. J. C. Lilly, *The Center of the Cyclone* (New York: Julian Press, 1972).

4. M. Vonnegut, *The Eden Express* (New York: Praeger, 1975), 81.

5. L. Schiller and A. Bennett, *The Quiet Room: A Journey Out of the Torment and Madness* (New York: Warner, 1994), 149–50.

6. M. Barnes and J. Berke, *Two Accounts of a Journey Through Madness* (New York: Harcout, Brace, Jovanovich, 1971), 69.

7. F. Dostoevsky, *The Idiot* (New York: Bantam Books, 1971), 218–19.

8. E. Thelmar, *The Maniac: A Realistic Study of Madness, From the Maniac's Point of View* (New York: American Psychical Institute, 1937), 258.

9. E. Thelmar, *The Maniac: A Realistic Study of Madness, From the Maniac's Point of View*, 257.

10. K. R. Jamison, *An Unquiet Mind: A Memoir of Moods and Madness* (New York: Knopf, 1995), 68.

11. T. Thompson, *The Beast: A Reckoning with Depression* (New York: G. P. Putnam's Sons, 1995), 217.

12. Alan Wheelis's book, *Quest for Identity* (New York: W. W. Norton, 1966), describes this basic existential dilemma well.

13. W. Styron, *Darkness Visible: A Memoir of Madness* (New York: Random House, 1990).

14. S. Plath, *The Bell Jar* (London: Faber and Faber, 1963), 168.

15. S. Plath, *The Bell Jar*, 170.

16. L. Wagner-Martin, *Sylvia Plath: A Biography* (New York: Simon and Schuster, 1987).

17. A. Boisen, *The Exploration of the Inner World, a Study of Mental Disorder and Religious Experience* (New York: Harper and Brothers, 1936 and 1952). Also see W. C. Alvarez, *Minds That Came Back* (Philadelphia: J. B. Lippincott, 1961), chapter 6.

18. V. Nijinsky, *The Diary of Vaslav Nijinsky* (London: Panther, 1963), 20.

19. V. Nijinsky, *The Diary of Vaslav Nijinsky*, 27.

20. J. Custance, "The Universe of Bliss and the Universe of Horror: A Description of a Manic-Depressive Psychosis," in B. Kaplan, ed., *The Inner World of Mental Illness* (New York: Harper and Row, 1964), 53.

21. H. E. Hughes, *The Man From Ida Grove: A Senator's Personal Story* (Lincoln, VA: Chosen Books, 1979), 87.

22. G. A. Miller, E. Galanter, and K. H. Pribram, *Plans and the Structure of Behavior* (New York: Holt, Rinehart and Winston, 1960).

23. See D. E. Rumelhart, P. Smolensky, J. L. McClelland, and G. E. Hinton, "Schemata and Sequential Thought Processes in PDP Models," in J. L. McClelland, D. E. Rumelhart, and the PDP Research Group (eds.), *Parallel Distributed Processing: Explorations in the Microstructure of Cognition, Volume 2: Psychological and Biological Models*, MIT Press, Cambridge, Massachusetts, 1986, 17–57; D. L. Reilly and L. N. Cooper, "An Overview of Neural Networks: Early Models to Real World Systems, in S. F. Zornetzer, J. L. Davis, and C. Lau, eds., *An Introduction to Neural and Electronic Networks*, Academic Press, New York, 1990, 227–48; and D. A. Norman, "Reflections on Cognition and Parallel Distributed Processing," in J. L. McClelland, D. E. Rumelhart, and the PDP Research Group, eds., *Parallel Distributed Processing,* 531–46.

24. J. L. Singer and P. Salovey, "Organized Knowledge Structures and Personality: Person Schemas, Self Schemas, Prototypes, and Scripts," in M. Horowitz, ed., *Person Schemas and Maladaptive Interpersonal Patterns* (Chicago: University of Chicago Press, 1991).

25. D. A. Norman, "Reflections on Cognition and Parallel Distributed Processing."

26. J. L. Singer and P. Salovey, "Organized Knowledge Structures and Personality: Person Schemas, Self Schemas, Prototypes, and Scripts."

27. See M. J. Horowitz, "Person Schemas," in M. J. Horowitz, ed., *Person Schemas and Maladaptive Interpersonal Patterns* (Chicago: University of Chicago Press, 1991).

28. D. R. Hofstadter, *Gödel, Escher, Bach: An Eternal Golden Braid* (New York: Vintage Books, 1980).

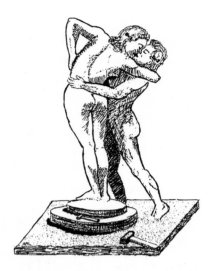

TEN: OTHER VERSIONS OF THE SELF

1. J. Kagan, *Galen's Prophesy: Temperament in Human Nature* (New York: Basic Books, 1994). Also see W. Gallagher, "How We Become What We Are," *The Atlantic Monthly*, September, 1994, 39–55; and C. R. Cloninger, D. M. Svrakic, and T. R. Przybeck, "A Psychological Model of Temperament and Character," *Archives of General Psychiatry*, 50 (1993): 975–90.

2. P. Packer, *Death of the Other Self* (New York: Cowles Book, 1970).

3. For representative approaches see M. Csikszentmihalyi, *The Evolving Self: A Psychology for the Third Millennium* (New York: HarperCollins, 1993); and C. Taylor, *The Ethics of Authenticity* (Cambridge: Harvard University Press, 1991).

4. R. J. Lifton, *The Protean Self: Human Resilience in an Age of Fragmentation* (New York: Basic Books, 1993).

5. See L. Rue, *By the Grace of Guile: The Role of Deception in Natural History and Human Affairs* (London: Oxford University Press, 1994).

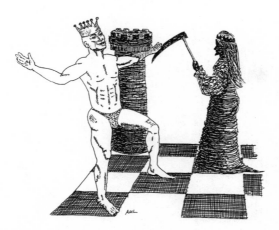

ELEVEN: BIOGRAPHICAL FREEDOM

1. See discussion in T. Honderich, *How Free Are You?: The Determinism Problem* (Oxford: Oxford University Press, 1993). Also see J. Trusted, *Freewill and Responsibility* (Oxford: Oxford University Press, 1984); B. F. Skinner, *Beyond Freedom and Dignity* (New York: Alfred A. Knopf, 1971); D. C. Dennett, *Elbow Room: The Varieties of Free Will Worth Wanting* (Oxford: Oxford University Press, 1984); S. Wolf, *Freedom Within Reason* (Oxford: Oxford University Press, 1990); and J. C. Eccles and K. Popper, *The Self and Its Brain* (New York: Springer International, 1977).

2. See S. E. Taylor, *Positive Illusions: Creative Self-Deception and the Healthy Mind* (New York: Basic Books, 1989).

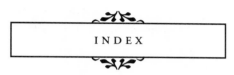

INDEX